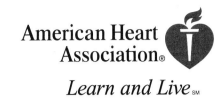

PALS
COURSE GUIDE

Editors

Mark Ralston, MD
  Oversight Editor
Mary Fran Hazinski, RN, MSN
  Senior Science Editor
Arno L. Zaritsky, MD
Stephen M. Schexnayder, MD
Monica E. Kleinman, MD

Special Contributors

Louis Gonzales, NREMT-P, *Senior Oversight Editor*
Brenda Drummonds, *PALS Writer*
Ulrik Christensen, MD
Frank Doto, MS, *Senior Oversight Editor*
Alan J. Schwartz, MD

American Academy of Pediatrics Reviewers

Susan Fuchs, MD
Wendy Simon, MA

PALS Subcommittee 2006-2007

Arno L. Zaritsky, MD, Chair
Stephen M. Schexnayder, MD, Immediate Past
  Chair, 2005-2006
Robert A. Berg, MD
Douglas S. Diekema, MD
Diana G. Fendya, RN, MSN
Mary Jo Grant, RN, PNP, PhD
George W. Hatch, Jr, EdD, EMT-P
Monica E. Kleinman, MD
Lester Proctor, MD
Faiqa A. Qureshi, MD
Ricardo A. Samson, MD
Elise W. van der Jagt, MD, MPH
Dianne L. Atkins, MD
Marc D. Berg, MD
Allan R. de Caen, MD
Michael J. Gerardi, MD
Jeffrey Perlman, MD
L. R. "Tres" Scherer III, MD, HSc
Wendy Simon, MA

ISBN 0-87493-527-X
© 2006 American Heart Association

i

To find out about any updates or corrections to this text, visit *www.americanheart.org/cpr* and click on the "Course Materials" button.

Contents

Student CD Contents

Contents

Part 1

Course Overview

Course Objectives

Introduction

The Pediatric Advanced Life Support (PALS) Provider Course is designed for healthcare providers who initiate and direct advanced life support beyond basic life support through the stabilization or transport phases of a pediatric emergency, either in or out of hospital. In this course you will enhance your skills in the evaluation and management of an infant or child with respiratory compromise, circulatory compromise, or cardiac arrest.

You will actively participate in a series of simulated core cases. These simulations are designed to reinforce important concepts, including

- identification and treatment of medical conditions that place the child at risk for cardiac arrest
- the systematic approach to pediatric assessment, including general assessment, primary assessment, secondary assessment, and tertiary assessment
- the assess-categorize-decide-act approach to assessment and management of a seriously ill infant or child
- PALS algorithms and flowcharts
- effective resuscitation team dynamics

The goal of the PALS Provider Course is to improve the quality of care provided to seriously ill or injured children, resulting in improved outcome.

Cognitive Course Objectives

Upon successful completion of this course, you should be able to

- understand and be able to perform the systematic approach to pediatric assessment of a seriously ill or injured child, including the general, primary, secondary, and tertiary assessments
- use the assess-categorize-decide-act approach to decision making
- recognize and manage a child in respiratory distress or failure and/or compensated or hypotensive shock
- recognize and manage a child with a life-threatening bradyarrhythmia, tachyarrhythmia, or arrest rhythm
- describe key elements of effective resuscitation team behaviors and explain why the foundation of successful resuscitation includes both mastery of basic skills and effective team dynamics
- prevent further deterioration of the child's condition during the stabilization and transfer phases of care

Psychomotor Course Objectives

At the end of the course you will be able to demonstrate the following skills:

- Performance of effective respiratory management skills, including use of oxygen delivery devices, suctioning, oropharyngeal airway (OPA), nasopharyngeal airway (NPA), bag-mask ventilation, and endotracheal (ET) intubation (according to scope of practice)
- Appropriate use of electrical therapy, including defibrillation and synchronized cardioversion
- Proper technique for intraosseous (IO) access and fluid bolus administration
- Performance as a team leader or team member in simulated cases

Course Description

Introduction

To help you achieve these objectives, the PALS Provider Course includes skills stations, CPR/AED competency testing, learning stations, core case testing stations, and a written test.

Skills Stations

The course includes the following skills stations:

- Management of Respiratory Emergencies
- Rhythm Disturbances/Electrical Therapy
- Vascular Access

During these stations you will have an opportunity to practice specific skills and then demonstrate competency. See the skills stations competency checklists in Part 3 for a listing of skills required in each station.

CPR/AED Competency Testing

Be prepared to pass the child 1-rescuer CPR/AED and the infant 1- and 2-rescuer CPR skills tests. *Make sure that you are proficient in BLS skills before attending the course.*

See Part 2: CPR/AED Competency Testing for testing requirements and resources.

Learning Stations

In the learning stations you will actively participate in a variety of learning activities, including

- core case discussions using a systematic approach to pediatric assessment and decision making
- core case simulations
- effective resuscitation team behaviors

In the learning stations you will apply your knowledge and practice essential skills both individually and as part of a team. This course emphasizes effective team skills as a vital part of the resuscitation effort. You will receive training in effective team behaviors and have the opportunity to practice as a team member and a team leader.

PALS Core Case Testing Stations

At the end of the course you will participate in 2 core case testing stations to validate your achievement of the course objectives. These simulated clinical scenarios will test the following:

- Knowledge of core case material and skills
- Management of respiratory and shock emergencies
- Management of rhythm disturbances, including interpretation of core arrhythmias and management with use of appropriate pharmacologic and electrical therapy
- Performance as a team leader

During the PALS core case testing stations you will be permitted to use the PALS pocket reference card and the ECC Handbook.

Written Test	The written test evaluates your mastery of the cognitive objectives. The written test is a closed-book test; no resources or aids are permitted. You must score 84% or better on the written test.

Course Materials

Introduction	Course materials consist of the *PALS Provider Manual*, student CD, and the *PALS Course Guide*.

Look for the following icons that direct you to these resources:

Icon	Course Material
	Student CD
	PALS Provider Manual

PALS Course Guide	The *PALS Course Guide* contains material that you will use *during the course* in the skills stations and learning stations. For example, you will use the skills station competency checklists as a guide to skills practice; your instructor will use these checklists to provide feedback. You will use the learning stations competency checklists in the case simulations and to prepare for the core case tests.

Remember to take this Course Guide with you to the course. |

Student CD	The student CD contains the self-assessment CD-based test, a vital part of your preparation for the course. Feedback from this assessment will help you identify gaps in your knowledge so that you can target specific material in the student CD and resource text to study.

Topic	Description	How to Use
Self-assessment CD-based test	Assessment consists of 3 parts: — ECG rhythm identification — pharmacology — practical application	Complete these assessments *before the course* to identify gaps in your knowledge

Topic	Description	How to Use
Practice cases	12 cases that illustrate the concepts of the pediatric assessment approach and "assess-categorize-decide-act" model	Read the cases and try to answer the questions. Check your answers to see if your responses are correct. Identify areas that need to be strengthened and improve your knowledge by studying the resource text, student CD, or other supplementary material.
Resuscitation team concept	Discusses the role of the team leader and team members; explains the 8 elements of effective team dynamics	Read before the course so that you are prepared to participate as a team member and team leader in case simulations and core case testing
Respiratory management resources	Resources and procedures for respiratory and circulatory management, eg, oxygen delivery systems, airway adjuncts, bag-mask ventilation, ET intubation	Review as necessary to prepare for the skills stations, case simulations, and core case tests; you must demonstrate competency in performance of skills according to your scope of practice
Vascular access procedures	IO and central venous access procedures	Review the IO access procedure to prepare for the vascular access skills station
Rhythm disturbances/electrical therapy procedures	Cardiac monitoring, synchronized cardioversion, manual defibrillation, and vagal maneuvers	Review these procedures to prepare for the rhythm disturbances/electrical therapy skills station, case simulations, and core case tests
ECG basics	Basic concepts of ECG interpretation	Review to prepare for the self-assessment CD-based test or use for remediation if you identify gaps in your knowledge
Pharmacology	Common drugs used in pediatric emergencies	
Safety and prevention	Scene assessment, sudden infant death syndrome (SIDS), sudden cardiac arrest (SCA)	Read to increase your knowledge of these topics

Topic	Description	How to Use
Ethical and legal aspects of CPR in children	Ethical and legal considerations of caring for critically ill children	Read to increase your knowledge of this topic
Chain of Survival	AHA Pediatric Chain of Survival illustrates a sequence of critical interventions to prevent death in children	Read to understand the shared responsibility of the community at large, caregivers, and healthcare professionals in saving children's lives

PALS Provider Manual

The *PALS Provider Manual* contains the information that you need to know to effectively participate in the course. This important material includes pediatric assessment concepts and recognition and management of respiratory, shock, and cardiac emergencies. *Please read and study this book before attending the course.* Some students may already know much of this information. Other students may need extensive study before the course.

The *PALS Provider Manual* is organized into the following chapters:

Chapter	Title	Content Summary
1	Pediatric Assessment	The systematic approach to pediatric assessment (general, primary, secondary, and tertiary assessments); the "assess-categorize-decide-act" model
2	Recognition of Respiratory Distress and Failure	Basic concepts of respiratory distress and failure and how to identify respiratory emergencies
3	Management of Respiratory Distress and Failure	Treatment options for respiratory emergencies
4	Recognition of Shock	Basic concepts of shock and how to identify compensated versus hypotensive shock
5	Management of Shock	Treatment options for shock
6	Recognition and Management of Bradyarrhythmias and Tachyarrhythmias	Recognition of clinical and ECG characteristics of bradyarrhythmias and tachyarrhythmias; medical and electrical therapies
7	Recognition and Management of Cardiac Arrest	Recognition of cardiac arrest by physical exam or arrest rhythm on the ECG monitor; medical and electrical therapy
8	Postresuscitation Management	Postresuscitation stabilization and transport
9	Pharmacology	Reference information on many common drugs used in pediatric emergencies

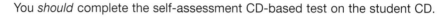

Precourse, Prerequisites, and Preparation

Precourse
Checklist

A precourse checklist accompanies this Course Guide. You must prepare for the course by doing all of the precourse work listed on the checklist. Without adequate preparation you may not successfully complete the course. Bring the completed checklist with you to the course.

This section discusses in detail each component listed on the precourse checklist.

Self-assessment
CD-based Test

You *should* complete the self-assessment CD-based test on the student CD.

Print your score and bring it with you to the course.

Course Prerequisites
and Preparation

Since the PALS Provider Course does not teach algorithms, ECG recognition, pharmacology, or CPR, complete the self-assessment CD-based test on the student CD to identify any gaps in your knowledge of these topics. The assessment will give you immediate feedback after each question and provide a summary of your strengths and weaknesses at the end. Use this information to identify any deficiencies in your knowledge. Increase your knowledge by studying applicable content in the *PALS Provider Manual,* Course Guide, the student CD, or other supplementary resources.

The following knowledge and skills are required for successful course completion:

- BLS skills
- ECG rhythm identification
- Basic pharmacology
- Practical application of knowledge to clinical scenarios
- Resuscitation team concepts

BLS Skills

Strong BLS skills are the foundation of advanced life support. It is essential that everyone who treats children and infants be able to perform high-quality CPR. Remember, whenever compressions are stopped, blood flow to the heart and brain stops, and drugs will not circulate. Patient survival often depends more on effective CPR than on advanced treatment. Without effective CPR for the victim of cardiac arrest, PALS interventions will fail. For this reason the PALS Provider Course requires that each student pass the child 1-rescuer CPR/AED and the infant 1- and 2-rescuer CPR skills tests. *Make sure that you are proficient in BLS skills before attending the course.*

See Part 2: CPR/AED Competency Testing for testing requirements and resources.

ECG Rhythm Identification

You must be able to identify and interpret these core rhythms during the case simulations and core case tests:

- Normal sinus rhythm
- Sinus bradycardia
- Sinus tachycardia
- Supraventricular tachycardia
- Ventricular tachycardia
- Ventricular fibrillation
- Asystole

The ECG rhythm identification section of the self-assessment CD-based test will help you evaluate your ability to identify these core rhythms as well as other common pediatric rhythms. If you have difficulty with pediatric rhythm identification, improve your knowledge by studying ECG Basics on the student CD, the *PALS Provider Manual*, Course Guide, or other supplementary resources.

Basic Pharmacology

You must know the basic pharmacology of the drugs used in the PALS algorithms and flow-charts. You will also need to know *when* to use *which* drug based on the clinical situation.

The pharmacology section of the self-assessment CD-based test will help you evaluate and enhance your knowledge of core drugs used in the course. You should know the indications, contraindications, and methods of administration. If you have difficulty with this section of the self-assessment, improve your knowledge by studying the *PALS Provider Manual*, student CD, Course Guide, and ECC Handbook.

Practical Application of Knowledge to Clinical Scenarios

The practical application section of the self-assessment CD-based test will help you evaluate your ability to apply your knowledge when presented with a clinical scenario. You will need to make decisions based on

- the pediatric assessment approach and the "assess-categorize-decide-act" model
- identification of core rhythms (if presented)
- knowledge of core drugs
- knowledge of PALS flowcharts and algorithms

Be sure that you understand pediatric assessment and "assess-categorize-decide-act" principles. Work through the practice cases on the student CD to identify weaknesses in your knowledge. Review the core rhythms and drugs. Be familiar with the PALS algorithms and flowcharts so that you can apply them to clinical scenarios. Note that the PALS course does not present the details of each algorithm. Sources of information are the *PALS Provider Manual*, the student CD, Course Guide, and the ECC Handbook.

Effective Resuscitation Team Concepts

Throughout the course you will be evaluated on your effectiveness as a team leader and a team member. In the core case tests you will be evaluated on your performance as a team leader. A major emphasis of this assessment will be your ability to direct the integration of BLS and PALS skills by your team members according to their scope of practice. Review Resuscitation Team Concept on the student CD before the course.

Requirements for Successful Course Completion

To successfully complete the PALS Provider Course and obtain your card, you must do the following:

- Actively participate in, practice, and complete all skills stations and learning stations
- Pass a skills test for child 1-rescuer CPR/AED and infant 1- and 2-rescuer CPR
- Pass a written test with a minimum score of 84%
- Pass 2 PALS core case tests as a team leader

Part 2

CPR/AED Competency Testing

Testing Requirements and Preparation

You must pass 2 CPR tests to receive a course completion card.

Skills Test Requirements
• Pass child 1-rescuer CPR/AED skills test
• Pass infant 1- and 2-rescuer CPR skills test

The PALS Provider Course does not include detailed instruction on how to do CPR or how to use an AED. You must know this in advance. Consider taking a BLS for Healthcare Providers Course if necessary. Review the student CPR practice sheets, Summary of BLS ABCD Maneuvers (Table 1), Pediatric BLS Algorithm (Figure 1), and CPR testing checklists in this part.

Student CPR Practice Sheets

Introduction

The child 1-rescuer CPR/AED student practice sheet and the infant 1- and 2-rescuer CPR student practice sheet provide detailed descriptions of the CPR skills that you will be expected to perform. Your instructor will evaluate your CPR skills during the skills test based on these descriptions.

If you perform a specific skill exactly as it is described in the critical performance step details, the instructor will check that specific skill as "passing." If you do not perform a specific skill exactly as it is described, the skill will not be checked off, and you will require remediation of that skill.

Study the following student CPR practice sheets so that you will be able to perform each skill correctly.

Child 1-Rescuer CPR/AED Student Practice Sheet

Step	Critical Performance Steps	Details
1	_____ Check for response	Tap victim and ask if the person is "all right" or "OK" speaking loudly and clearly.
2	_____ Activate the emergency response system: Tell someone to phone 911 and get an AED	Activate the emergency response system by making sure that someone phones 911 and gets an AED.
3	_____ Open airway using head tilt–chin lift	Place palm of one hand on forehead and push the head back. Place fingers of other hand under the lower jaw to lift the chin. Do not completely close mouth. Move the head back toward the hand on the forehead in a way that is clearly visible to the instructor.
4	_____ Check for breathing	Place face near the victim's nose and mouth. Look at chest and listen and feel for breathing. Continue for at least 5 seconds but no more than 10 seconds.
5	_____ Give 2 breaths (1 second each) that produce visible chest rise	Use a pocket mask, seal mask around mouth and nose, and give breaths. Give each rescue breath over approximately 1 second. Reposition the head if chest does not rise. You may make multiple attempts to reposition head or improve seal to give breaths that make the chest rise. You should give 2 breaths that produce visible chest rise. Take no more than 10 seconds to accomplish 2 breaths, then move to compressions.
6	_____ Check for carotid pulse	Place two or three fingers on the trachea and slip the fingers into the groove between the trachea and muscles on the side of the neck. Check for pulse for at least 5 seconds but no more than 10 seconds.
7	_____ Locate CPR hand position	Move or remove clothing from victim's chest. Place heel of one hand in the center of chest between the nipples. You may place the other hand on top of the first hand (if needed to compress the chest to the correct depth). Extend or interlace fingers to keep off chest.
8	_____ Deliver first cycle of 30 compressions at the correct rate	Keep hand(s) in proper place on chest. Give 30 compressions in less than 23 seconds. Push hard, push fast; allow chest to return to normal between compressions.

Step	Critical Performance Steps	Details
9	_____ Give 2 breaths (1 second each) with visible chest rise	Use a pocket mask, seal mask around mouth and nose, and give breaths.
		Give each rescue breath over approximately 1 second.
		Reposition the head if chest does not rise.
		You may make multiple attempts to reposition head or improve seal to give breaths that make the chest rise.
		You should give 2 breaths that produce visible chest rise.
		Take no more than 10 seconds to accomplish 2 breaths, then move to compressions.
AED Arrives		
AED 1	_____ Turn AED on	Stop CPR and press button to turn AED on (or make sure that AED case is open if your AED has an automatic-on feature).
AED 2	_____ Select proper pads and place pads correctly	You must recognize the difference between adult pads and child pads, select the proper pad size for the child victim, and apply the pads to the chest as illustrated on the pads and/or AED instructions.
AED 3	_____ Clear victim to allow AED to analyze rhythm	Show a visible sign of clearing the victim along with a verbal indication of clearing the victim: "Clear! Stay clear of victim!" or similar statement with an obvious gesture to ensure that all are clear.
AED 4	_____ Clear victim to deliver shock/ Press shock button	Show a visible sign of clearing the victim along with a verbal indication of clearing the victim: "Clear! Stay clear of victim!" or similar statement with an obvious gesture to ensure that all are clear.
		Press shock button when prompted and after clearing.
10	_____ Resume CPR: deliver second cycle of 30 compressions using correct hand position	Resume CPR, beginning with compressions, immediately after shock delivery. Place heel of one hand in the center of chest, between the nipples.
		You may place the other hand on top of the first hand (if needed to compress the chest to the correct depth).
		Extend or interlace fingers to keep off chest.
		Do 30 compressions.
11	_____ Give 2 breaths (1 second each) that produce visible chest rise	Use a pocket mask, seal mask around mouth and nose, and give breaths.
		Give each rescue breath over approximately 1 second.
		Reposition the head if chest does not rise.
		You may make multiple attempts to reposition head or improve seal to give breaths that make the chest rise.
		You should give 2 breaths that produce visible chest rise.
		Take no more than 10 seconds to accomplish 2 breaths and then move to compressions.
12	_____ Deliver third cycle of 30 compressions of adequate depth with chest returning to normal position after each compression	Push hard, push fast; allow chest to return to normal between compressions.
		You must do at least 23 of 30 compressions correctly: adequate depth and allowing the chest to return to normal between compressions.

Infant 1- and 2-Rescuer CPR Student Practice Sheet

Step	Critical Performance Steps	Details
1	_____ Check for response	Tap infant and shout loudly.
2	_____ Activate emergency response system	Tell bystander to activate appropriate emergency response.
3	_____ Open airway using head tilt–chin lift	Push back on manikin forehead; place fingers of other hand on the bony part of the victim's chin, and lift the victim's chin. Do not press the soft tissues of the neck or under the chin. Lift the jaw upward by bringing the chin forward. Do NOT hyperextend the neck.
4	_____ Check for breathing	Place face near the victim's nose and mouth. Look at chest and listen and feel for breathing. Continue for at least 5 seconds but no more than 10 seconds.
5	_____ Give 2 breaths (1 second each) that produce visible chest rise	Use a pocket mask, seal mask around mouth and nose, and give breaths. Give each rescue breath over approximately 1 second. Reposition the head if chest does not rise. You may make multiple attempts to reposition head or improve seal to give breaths that make the chest rise. You should give 2 breaths that produce visible chest rise. Take no more than 10 seconds to accomplish 2 breaths, then move to compressions.
6	_____ Check for brachial pulse	Locate the brachial pulse in the manikin's upper arm closer to you, using the fingers to try to feel the pulse between the biceps muscle and the humerus. Gently feel for a pulse for at least 5 seconds but no more than 10 seconds.
7	_____ Locate CPR finger position	Place 2 fingers on the sternum just below the nipple line.
8	_____ Deliver first cycle of 30 compressions at the correct rate	Give 30 compressions in less than 23 seconds. Push hard, push fast; allow chest to return to normal position between compressions.
9	_____ Give 2 breaths (1 second each) that produce visible chest rise	Use a pocket mask, seal mask around mouth and nose, and give breaths. Give each rescue breath over approximately 1 second. Reposition the head if chest does not rise. You should give 2 breaths that produce visible chest rise. Take no more than 10 seconds to accomplish 2 breaths, then move to compressions.

Step	Critical Performance Steps	Details
	Second rescuer will help perform CPR, taking over rescue breaths, using a bag mask. Rescuers should use a 15:2 compression–to–ventilation ratio.	
10	_____ Deliver cycle of 15 compressions using 2 thumb–encircling hands technique	Compress lower half of sternum with 2 thumb–encircling hands technique in proper position. Squeeze hands while compressing with thumbs. Do 15 compressions.
11	_____ Pause to allow 2nd rescuer to give 2 breaths	Pause compressions to allow 2nd rescuer to give 2 breaths with bag mask.
12	_____ Deliver cycle of 15 compressions of adequate depth with full chest recoil	Push hard, push fast; allow full chest recoil between compressions. Do 15 compressions.
13	_____ Pause to allow 2nd rescuer to give 2 breaths	Pause compressions to allow 2nd rescuer to give 2 breaths with bag mask.
	Switch places with little interruption. You take over rescue breaths, using bag mask. Two more CPR cycles are performed.	
14	_____ Give 2 breaths that produce visible chest rise during pauses in compressions using bag mask (2 cycles)	Use bag mask, seal mask properly, and squeeze bag. Two breaths should produce visible chest rise. Breaths should take approximately 1 second each. You may make multiple attempts to reposition head or improve seal to give breaths that make the chest rise. (Sounds of an air leak can be present as long as there is visible chest rise.) Repeat for 2 cycles with 2nd rescuer doing chest compressions.

Remediation

Remediation Lesson   Any student who does not pass both skills tests will practice and be remediated during the Remediation Lesson at the end of the course.

Students who need remediation testing will be tested in the *entire* skill.

Summary of BLS

Introduction   Review the summary of BLS steps for all pediatric ages in Table 1. Remember that for healthcare providers, guidelines are specific to the age of the child and are as follows:

- Child guidelines for CPR apply to age 1 year to adolescent (defined by onset of puberty)
- Child guidelines for use of an AED with a pediatric attenuated defibrillation dose apply to age 1 year to age 8 years

Table 1. Summary of BLS ABCD Maneuvers for Infants, Children, and Adults

(Newborn/Neonatal information not included) *Note:* Maneuvers used only by healthcare providers are indicated by "HCP."

Maneuver	Adult Lay rescuer: ≥8 years HCP: Adolescent and older	Child Lay rescuers: 1 to 8 years HCP: 1 year to adolescent	Infant Under 1 year of age
ACTIVATE Emergency Response Number (lone rescuer)	Activate when victim found unresponsive **HCP:** if asphyxial arrest likely, call after 5 cycles (2 minutes) of CPR	Activate after performing 5 cycles of CPR For sudden, witnessed collapse, activate after verifying that victim unresponsive	
AIRWAY	Head tilt–chin lift (HCP: suspected trauma, use jaw thrust)		
BREATHS Initial	2 breaths at 1 second/breath	2 effective breaths at 1 second/breath	
HCP: Rescue breathing without chest compressions	10 to 12 breaths/min (approximately 1 breath every 5 to 6 seconds)	12 to 20 breaths/min (approximately 1 breath every 3 to 5 seconds)	
HCP: Rescue breaths for CPR with advanced airway	8 to 10 breaths/min (approximately 1 breath every 6 to 8 seconds)		
Foreign-body airway obstruction	Abdominal thrusts		Back slaps and chest thrusts
CIRCULATION **HCP:** Pulse check (≤10 sec)	Carotid (**HCP** can use femoral in child)		Brachial or femoral
Compression landmarks	Center of chest, between nipples		Just below nipple line
Compression method Push hard and fast Allow complete recoil	**2 Hands:** Heel of 1 hand, other hand on top	**2 Hands:** Heel of 1 hand with second on top or **1 Hand:** Heel of 1 hand only	1 rescuer: 2 fingers **HCP**, 2 rescuers: 2 thumb–encircling hands
Compression depth	1½ to 2 inches	Approximately ⅓ to ½ the depth of the chest	
Compression rate	Approximately 100/min		
Compression-ventilation ratio	30:2 (1 or 2 rescuers)	30:2 (single rescuer) **HCP:** 15:2 (2 rescuers)	
DEFIBRILLATION			
AED	Use adult pads. Do not use child pads/child system. **HCP:** For out-of-hospital response may provide 5 cycles/2 minutes of CPR before shock if response > 4 to 5 minutes and arrest not witnessed.	**HCP:** Use AED as soon as available for sudden collapse and in-hospital. **All:** After about 2 minutes of CPR (out-of-hospital). Use child pads/child system for child 1 to 8 years if available. If child pads/system not available, use adult AED and pads.	No recommendation for infants <1 year of age

Pediatric BLS for Healthcare Providers Algorithm

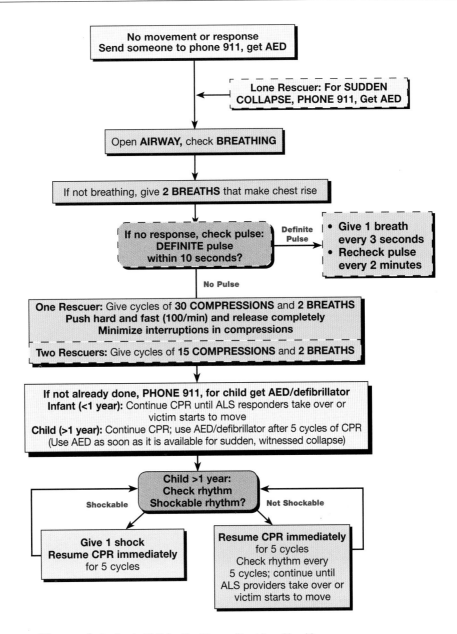

Figure 1. Pediatric BLS for Healthcare Providers Algorithm

PALS CPR Testing Checklist

Introduction

The instructor will record your skills tests results on the CPR testing checklist:

- The first page of the checklist is for the child CPR + AED skills test.
- The second page is for the infant 1- and 2-rescuer CPR skills test.

Review the CPR testing checklist to understand the criteria your instructor will use to evaluate your skills.

PALS CPR Testing Checklist

American Heart Association **PEDIATRIC ADVANCED LIFE SUPPORT** Child 1-Rescuer CPR and AED Test	Name: _____ Date of Test: _____

Skill Step	Child 1-Rescuer CPR With AED C R I T I C A L P E R F O R M A N C E S T E P S	☑ if done correctly
1	Checks for response	
2	Activates the emergency response system: Tells someone to phone 911 and get an AED	
3	Opens airway using head tilt–chin lift	
4	Checks for breathing *Minimum 5 seconds; maximum 10 seconds*	
5	Gives 2 breaths (1 second each) that produce visible chest rise	
6	Checks for carotid pulse *Minimum 5 seconds; maximum 10 seconds*	
7	Locates CPR hand position	
8	Delivers first cycle of 30 compressions at correct rate *Acceptable <23 seconds for 30 compressions*	
9	Gives 2 breaths (1 second each) that produce visible chest rise	
AED Arrives.		
AED 1	Turns AED On	
AED 2	Selects proper AED pads and places pads correctly	
AED 3	Clears victim to analyze *(Must be visible and verbal check)*	
AED 4	Clears victim to shock/Presses shock button *(Must be visible and verbal check) Maximum time from AED arrival <90 sec*	
Student continues CPR.		
10	Delivers second cycle of 30 compressions at correct hand position *Acceptable >23 of 30 compressions at correct position*	
11	Gives 2 breaths (1 second each) with visible chest rise	
The next step is done only with a manikin with a feedback device, such as a clicker or light. If not, STOP THE TEST.		
12	Delivers third cycle of 30 compressions of adequate depth with full chest recoil *Acceptable >23 comps of 30 with adequate depth and recoil*	

CPR TEST RESULTS	Indicate Pass or Needs Remediation	CPR/AED		INFANT		STOP THE TEST	
		P	NR	P	NR	P	NR
INST SIGNATURE:							

American Heart Association **PEDIATRIC ADVANCED LIFE SUPPORT** Infant 1- and 2-Rescuer CPR Test	Name: _____ Date of Test: _____

Skill Step	Infant 1- and 2-Rescuer CPR C R I T I C A L P E R F O R M A N C E S T E P S	☑ if done correctly
1	**Checks for response**	
2	**Activates emergency response system**	
3	**Opens airway using head tilt–chin lift**	
4	**Checks for breathing** *Minimum 5 seconds; maximum 10 seconds*	
5	**Gives 2 breaths (1 second each) that produce visible chest rise**	
6	**Checks for brachial pulse** *Minimum 5 seconds; maximum 10 seconds*	
7	**Locates CPR finger position**	
8	**Delivers first cycle of 30 compressions at correct rate** *Acceptable <23 seconds for 30 compressions*	
9	**Gives 2 breaths (1 second each) with visible chest rise**	
Second rescuer arrives and takes over breathing with bag mask. Test only first rescuer. Rescuers use 15:2 ratio.		
10	**1st rescuer delivers cycle of 15 compressions using 2 thumb–encircling hands technique** *Acceptable >11 of 15 compressions at correct position*	
11	**1st rescuer pauses to allow 2nd rescuer to give 2 breaths**	
12	**1st rescuer delivers cycle of 15 compressions of adequate depth with full chest recoil** *Measure depth only if using instrumented manikin; otherwise observe that compressions are given.*	
13	**1st rescuer pauses to allow 2nd rescuer to give 2 breaths**	
Rescuers switch places with little interruption. 1st rescuer takes over rescue breaths using bag mask. Students perform 2 more cycles of CPR. Test only 1st rescuer.		
14	**1st rescuer gives 2 breaths that produce visible chest rise during pauses in compressions using bag mask (2 cycles)**	

STOP THE TEST	
P	NR

Mark results for this test on bottom of other side

Part 3

Skills Stations

Overview

In the skills stations you will practice and demonstrate competency in specific resuscitation skills, such as bag-mask ventilation and establishing IO access. Skills stations in the PALS Provider Course are:

- Management of Respiratory Emergencies
- Rhythm Disturbances/Electrical Therapy
- Vascular Access

Use the checklists at the end of this part to prepare for these skills stations. Review the steps on the checklists and study applicable procedures in Respiratory Management Resources and Vascular Access Procedures on the student CD.

Refer to the checklists during the course while practicing the skills. Your instructor will evaluate your skills based on the criteria specified in these checklists.

Management of Respiratory Emergencies Skills Station

Station Overview

In the management of respiratory emergencies skills station you will have an opportunity to practice and demonstrate competency in airway management skills.

Station Objectives

In this station you will demonstrate

- insertion of OPA; knowledge of indications and method for insertion of an NPA
- effective bag-mask ventilation
- OPA and ET tube suctioning
- confirmation of ET tube placement by physical exam and by using an exhaled CO_2 detection device
- securing the ET tube

If it is within your scope of practice, you will demonstrate advanced airway skills, including correct insertion of an ET tube and placement of a nasogastric (NG)/orogastric (OG) tube for gastric decompression.

Rhythm Disturbances/Electrical Therapy Skills Station

Station Overview

In the rhythm disturbances/electrical therapy skills station you will have an opportunity to practice and demonstrate competency in rhythm identification and operation of a cardiac monitor and manual defibrillator.

Station Objectives

In this skills station you will demonstrate

- correct placement of ECG leads
- correct paddle/electrode pad selection and positioning
- identification of rhythms that require defibrillation
- identification of rhythms that require synchronized cardioversion
- operation of a cardiac monitor
- safe performance of manual defibrillation and synchronized cardioversion

Vascular Access Skills Station

Station Overview

In the vascular access skills station you will have an opportunity to practice and demonstrate competency in IO access and other vascular access skills.

Station Objectives

In this skills station you will

- insert an IO needle
- summarize how to confirm that the needle has reached the marrow cavity
- summarize/demonstrate the method of giving an IV/IO bolus
- use a length-based/color-coded resuscitation tape to calculate correct drug doses
- (optional) establish (IV) access

Skills Station Competency Checklists

Management of Respiratory Emergencies Skills Station Competency Checklist

Critical Performance Steps	☑ if done correctly
Verbalizes difference between high-flow and low-flow O$_2$ delivery systems • High flow (>10 L/min): O$_2$ flow exceeds patient inspiratory flow, preventing entrainment of room air if system is tight-fitting; delivers up to 0.95 FiO$_2$, eg, nonrebreathing mask with reservoir • Low flow (≤10 L/min): patient inspiratory flow exceeds O$_2$ flow, allowing entrainment of room air; delivers 0.23 to 0.80 FiO$_2$, eg, nasal cannula, simple O$_2$ mask	
Verbalizes maximum nasal cannula flow rate (4 L/min)	
Opens airway using head tilt–chin lift maneuver while keeping mouth open (jaw thrust for trauma victim)	
Verbalizes different indications for OPA and NPA • OPA only for unconscious victim without a gag reflex • NPA for conscious or semiconscious victim	
Selects correctly sized airway by measuring • OPA from corner of mouth to angle of mandible • NPA from tip of nose to tragus of ear	
Inserts OPA correctly	
Looks, listens, feels for breathing after OPA insertion	
Suctions with OPA in place; states suctioning not to exceed 10 seconds	
Selects correct mask size for ventilations	
Applies bag-mask device and opens airway using E-C clamp technique	
Gives 2 breaths (1 second each) causing chest rise with bag-mask device	
All students must demonstrate the following steps.	
States equipment needed for endotracheal (ET) tube intubation procedure	
Confirms proper ET tube placement by physical exam and by using an exhaled CO$_2$ device	
Secures ET tube	
Suctions with ET tube in place	
The following steps are optional. They are demonstrated and evaluated only when the student's scope of practice involves endotracheal intubation.	
Prepares equipment for ET intubation	
Inserts ET tube correctly	
Places or describes placement of NG/OG tube for gastric decompression	

Rhythm Disturbances/Electrical Therapy Skills Station Competency Checklist

Critical Performance Steps	☑ if done correctly
Applies ECG leads correctly • White lead: to right shoulder • Red lead: to left ribs, flank • Black, green or brown lead: to left shoulder	
Demonstrates correct operation of monitor: • Turns monitor on • Adjusts device to manual mode (not AED mode) to display rhythm in standard limb leads (I, II, III) or paddles/electrode pads	
Verbalizes correct electrical therapy for appropriate core rhythms: • Synchronized cardioversion for unstable SVT, VT with pulses • Defibrillation for pulseless VT, VF	
Makes correct paddle/electrode pad selection for infant or child; places paddles/ electrode pads in correct position	
Demonstrates correct and safe synchronized cardioversion • Places device in synchronized mode • Selects appropriate energy (0.5-1 J/kg) • Charges, clears, delivers current	
Demonstrates correct and safe manual defibrillation • Places device in unsynchronized mode • Selects energy (2-4 J/kg) • Charges, clears, delivers current	

Vascular Access Skills Station Competency Checklist

Critical Performance Steps	☑ if done correctly
Verbalizes indications for IO insertion	
Verbalizes sites for IO insertion (anterior tibia, distal femur, medial malleolus, anterior superior iliac spine)	
Verbalizes contraindications for IO placement • Fracture in extremity • Previous insertion attempt in extremity that entered marrow space • Infection overlying bone	
Inserts IO catheter safely	
Verbalizes how to confirm IO catheter is in correct position; verbalizes how to secure IO catheter	
Attaches IV line to IO catheter; demonstrates giving IO fluid bolus using 3-way stopcock and syringe	
Shows how to determine correct drug doses using a length-based/color-coded tape or other resource	
The following is optional:	
Verbalizes correct procedure for establishing IV access	

Part 4

Pediatric Assessment

Systematic Approach to Pediatric Assessment

General Assessment

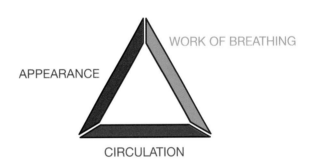

The general assessment is a visual and auditory assessment of the child's general appearance during the first few seconds of encounter. The pediatric assessment triangle (PAT) is a reminder to evaluate the *appearance, work of breathing,* and *circulation.*

> *If you recognize a life-threatening condition at any time, immediately begin life-saving interventions and activate the emergency response system (ERS).*

If the general assessment does not reveal a life-threatening condition requiring immediate intervention, proceed with the primary assessment.

Primary Assessment

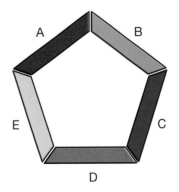

The primary assessment is a rapid hands-on ABCDE evaluation of cardiopulmonary and neurologic function. This assessment includes vital signs and oxygen saturation by pulse oximetry.

Airway	Assess airway to decide if it is patent. Determine if you can open and maintain the airway with simple measures (eg, positioning, head tilt–chin lift, suctioning, techniques to relieve foreign-body airway obstruction [FBAO], airway adjuncts) or if you need advanced interventions (ET intubation, removal of foreign body, cricothyrotomy, NPA placement, or continuous positive airway pressure [CPAP]).
Breathing	To assess breathing, evaluate • respiratory rate • respiratory effort • tidal volume • airway and lung sounds • oxyhemoglobin saturation by pulse oximetry Note whether the inspiratory or expiratory phase (or both) is affected.
Circulation	Assess circulation by evaluating both cardiovascular and end-organ function. Evaluate cardiovascular function by assessing • skin color and temperature • heart rate and rhythm • pulses (both peripheral and central) • capillary refill time • blood pressure, including pulse pressure Evaluate end-organ function by assessing • brain perfusion (mental status) • skin perfusion • renal perfusion (urine output)
Disability	Assess disability to establish the child's level of consciousness. Standard evaluations are • AVPU pediatric response scale • Glasgow Coma Scale (GCS) • pupillary responses
Exposure	Remove clothing as necessary to look for evidence of trauma (eg, burns, bruising, bleeding). Palpate the extremities to assess for injury. Measure core temperature. Keep the child warm to prevent hypothermia. Note: Use spine precautions when turning any patient with suspected spine injury.

Secondary Assessment

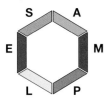

The secondary assessment consists of a focused medical history using the SAMPLE mnemonic and a thorough physical examination. SAMPLE stands for

- **S**igns and **S**ymptoms
- **A**llergies
- **M**edications
- **P**ast medical history
- **L**ast meal
- **E**vents leading to presentation

Tertiary Assessment

The tertiary assessment includes laboratory, radiographic, and other advanced tests to help establish the child's physiologic condition and diagnosis. The term *tertiary* does not mean these tests are performed third. The timing of tertiary tests is dictated by the clinical situation.

Resources

You must have a thorough understanding of the systematic approach to pediatric assessment to participate effectively in the core case discussions, core case simulations, and core case testing stations in the PALS Provider Course. Be sure to complete the self-assessment CD-based test several days before the course to identify areas where you need to increase your knowledge. Review the Pediatric Assessment chapter in the Provider Manual. Validate your understanding by working through some of the practice cases on the student CD and checking your answers.

Assess, Categorize, Decide, and Act

Introduction

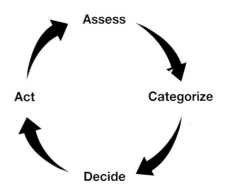

During the case discussions and case simulations, you will practice the "assess-categorize-decide-act" approach to the assessment and management of a seriously ill or injured child. This is an iterative process that is repeated frequently during evaluation and management.

Remember that if you recognize a life-threatening condition at any time, begin life-saving interventions immediately and activate the ERS.

Assess

Assess and reassess using the systematic approach to pediatric assessment. Begin your evaluation of the child using the general assessment (PAT) and the primary assessment. Proceed with the secondary and tertiary assessments after appropriate interventions are initiated to stabilize the child.

Categorize

Attempt to categorize the clinical condition by type and severity:

	Type	**Severity**
Respiratory	• Upper airway obstruction • Lower airway obstruction • Lung tissue (parenchymal) disease • Disordered control of breathing	• Respiratory distress • Respiratory failure
Circulatory	• Hypovolemic shock • Obstructive shock • Distributive/septic shock • Cardiogenic shock	• Compensated shock • Hypotensive shock

The clinical condition can also be a combination of respiratory and circulatory problems. As the child deteriorates, one category of problems may lead to others.

Note that in the initial phase of your evaluation you may be uncertain about the type or severity of problems, or both.

Decide

Based on your assessment and categorization of the condition, decide appropriate management based on your scope of practice.

Act

Start treatment interventions appropriate for the clinical condition.

Resources

Please read and study the Pediatric Assessment chapter in the Provider Manual. Work through the practice cases on the student CD.

*If you recognize a life-threatening condition at any time,
immediately begin life-saving interventions and activate the ERS.*

Pediatric Assessment Flowchart

Introduction

Figure 2 outlines the systematic approach to pediatric assessment.

- Conduct a visual and auditory assessment of the general appearance in the first few seconds of patient encounter.
- Evaluate the ABCDEs during the primary assessment.
- Proceed with the secondary and tertiary assessment once the child's condition has been stabilized.

Throughout your evaluation, look for life-threatening conditions. If you identify one, intervene immediately and activate the ERS.

General Assessment
Appearance ▲ Work of Breathing ▲ Circulation

Primary Assessment
Airway Breathing Circulation Disability Exposure

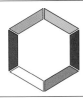

Secondary Assessment
(SAMPLE history, focused
physical exam, bedside glucose)

Tertiary Assessment
(laboratory studies, x-rays, other tests)

Categorize illness by type and severity

Respiratory	Circulatory
Respiratory distress *or* *Respiratory failure*	*Compensated shock* *or* *Hypotensive shock*
Upper airway obstruction Lower airway obstruction Lung tissue disease Disordered control of breathing	Hypovolemic shock Distributive shock Cardiogenic shock Obstructive shock

Respiratory   +   Circulatory
including cardiopulmonary failure

If at any time during the assessment and categorization process you identify a life-threatening condition

Immediately initiate life-saving interventions

and

activate the emergency response system

Figure 2. Pediatric Assessment Flowchart

Life-threatening Conditions

Recognition

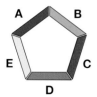

Be alert to life-threatening conditions, such as the following:

Airway	Complete or severe airway obstruction
Breathing	Apnea, significant work of breathing, bradypnea
Circulation	Absence of detectable pulses, poor perfusion, hypotension, bradycardia
Disability	Unresponsiveness, depressed consciousness
Exposure	Significant hypothermia, significant bleeding, petechiae consistent with septic shock, abdominal distention consistent with an acute abdomen

Interventions

If you recognize a life-threatening condition, begin life-saving interventions. Examples of these interventions are

- support ABCs (CPR for cardiac arrest)
- provide supplementary 100% oxygen
- provide assisted ventilation, eg, bag-mask, ET intubation
- start cardiac and respiratory monitoring, eg, ECG, pulse oximetry, exhaled CO_2 if intubated
- establish IV/IO access
- give a bolus of isotonic crystalloid
- obtain laboratory studies such as bedside glucose and arterial blood gas (ABG)
- administer drugs
- provide electrical therapy

Resuscitation Team Concept

Effective Team Dynamics

Introduction

Successful teams not only have medical expertise and mastery of resuscitation skills but also demonstrate effective communication and team dynamics. The PALS Provider Course stresses the importance of team roles and effective team dynamics.

During the course you will have an opportunity to practice different roles of a simulated resuscitation team, including the role of a team leader.

Observe 8 Elements

Look for opportunities during the case simulations to practice and observe the following 8 elements of effective team dynamics. Make notes of examples (positive and negative) that you observe during the course.

Table 2. Effective Team Dynamics Observation Sheet

	Element	Observed
1	Closed-loop communication	
2	Clear messages	
3	Clear roles and responsibilities	
4	Knowing one's limitations	
5	Knowledge sharing	

	Element	Observed
6	Constructive intervention	
7	Reevaluation and summarizing	
8	Mutual respect	

Summary of Team Roles

Roles and Responsibilities

During the course *each* student will have an opportunity to participate in the following team roles:

Role	Responsibilities
Team leader	• Directs the resuscitation • Monitors performance of tasks • Models excellent team behavior
Airway	• Checks oxygen setup • Administers oxygen • Inserts OPA or NPA • Performs bag-mask ventilation • Inserts NG/OG tube • Prepares/performs ET intubation (based on scope of practice)
IV/IO	• Gains IV/IO access • Prepares drugs and fluids • Administers drugs and fluids
Compressor	• Performs chest compressions • If chest compressions are not needed during a case, team member may obtain equipment, fluids, and drugs or assist the observer/recorder
Monitor/ defibrillator	• Establishes ECG monitoring • Checks pulse • Operates monitor/defibrillator
Observer/recorder	• Monitors performance of the team using the learning stations competency checklist

See Figure 3 for location of team members during case simulations.

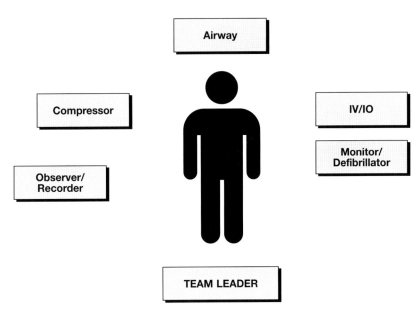

Figure 3. Suggested locations for the team leader and team members during the case simulations.

Cardiac Arrest

Recognition of Cardiac Arrest

Introduction

Cardiac arrest is the cessation of blood circulation (flow) as a result of absent or ineffective cardiac mechanical activity. Signs of circulation are absent. Cerebral hypoxia causes victims to lose consciousness and stop breathing, although agonal gasps may be present in the first seconds after a sudden cardiac arrest.

Pediatric cardiac arrest is uncommon. In contrast to cardiac arrest in adults, cardiac arrest in children is rarely *sudden cardiac arrest* caused by primary cardiac arrhythmias. Cardiac arrest in children is most often *asphyxial*, resulting from the progression of respiratory distress and failure or shock, or both (Figure 4).

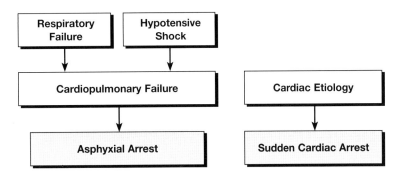

Figure 4. Pathway to cardiac arrest

Whereas outcomes from respiratory distress and failure, respiratory arrest, or shock in children are generally good, outcomes from pediatric cardiac arrest are generally poor. Focus on prevention of cardiac arrest by

- preventing disease processes that lead to cardiac arrest
- early recognition and management of respiratory distress and failure, respiratory arrest, and shock before deterioration to cardiac arrest

Clinical Signs and Rhythms

Cardiac arrest is recognized by clinical signs and by specific rhythms.

Clinical signs of cardiac arrest are

- apnea or agonal gasps
- no palpable pulses
- unresponsiveness

Since the accuracy of a pulse check is poor, recognition of cardiac arrest may be determined by the *absence* of clinical signs of life, including the absence of adequate breathing (other than agonal gasps), coughing, or movement in response to stimulation.

Rhythms associated with pulseless arrest are

- pulseless ventricular tachycardia (VT)
- ventricular fibrillation (VF)
- asystole

Importance of High-Quality BLS

Introduction

High-quality CPR is the foundation of basic and advanced life support for the management of cardiac arrest. Until the defibrillator arrives, a team member should perform immediate high-quality CPR.

High-Quality CPR

The following are characteristics of good chest compressions:

Push hard	• Push with sufficient force to depress the chest approximately one third to one half the anterior/posterior diameter • *Release completely,* allowing the chest to fully recoil
Push fast	Push at a rate of approximately 100 compressions per minute
Minimize interruptions	• Try to limit interruptions in chest compressions to 10 seconds or less or as needed for interventions (eg, defibrillation or insertion of an advanced airway). Ideally compressions are interrupted only for ventilation (until an advanced airway is placed), rhythm check, and actual shock delivery. • Once an advanced airway is in place, you will no longer perform "cycles" of CPR (compressions paused for breaths). Rescuers will provide continuous ventilations (ie, 8 to 10 breaths per minute) and continuous chest compressions (100/minute) ideally interrupted only by rhythm check and shock delivery.

Chest compressions should ideally be interrupted only for ventilation (until an advanced airway is placed), rhythm check, and actual shock delivery.

Sequence of Actions Based on Likely Cause of Arrest

Prioritize management based on the likely cause of the arrest.

If the arrest is	Then...
Unwitnessed (assumed to be asphyxial in origin) in the out-of-hospital setting	• Start immediate CPR • Perform cycles of chest compressions and ventilations for about 2 minutes • Apply AED and follow prompts
Witnessed (sudden collapse more likely to be cardiac in origin) and in-hospital arrest	• Send someone to activate the ERS and get an AED/defibrillator while you begin CPR. If you are alone, you must activate the ERS and then begin the steps of CPR. • Apply the AED (and follow voice prompts) or manual defibrillator as soon as one is available for a child who is unresponsive, not breathing, with no pulse.

Summary

Remember that even the best advanced life support interventions will be ineffective if BLS is of poor quality.

Resources

Read the Recognition and Management of Cardiac Arrest chapter in the Provider Manual.

Rhythm Strips: Arrest Rhythms

Introduction

You must be able to identify arrest rhythms (ie, pulseless VT, VF, asystole) during the course. Study the following rhythm strips to prepare for the rhythm disturbances/electrical therapy skills stations, the case simulations, and the core case tests.

Pulseless VT (Monomorphic)

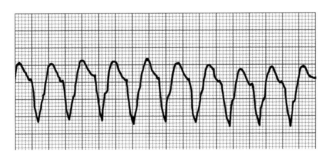

Figure 5. Pulseless ventricular tachycardia (monomorphic).

VF

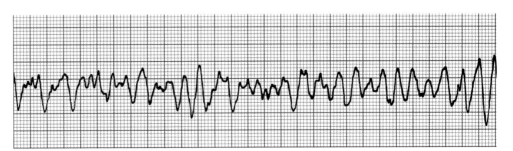

Figure 6. Ventricular fibrillation.

Organized Rhythm Returns After Defibrillation

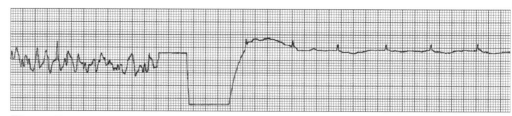

Figure 7. Organized rhythm returns after defibrillation.

Asystole

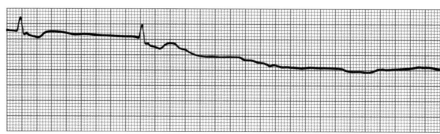

Figure 8. Asystole from initial bradyarrhythmia.

PALS Pulseless Arrest Algorithm

Introduction

Study the PALS Pulseless Arrest Algorithm (Figure 9) to prepare for the course. You will be presented with pulseless arrest scenarios during the rhythm disturbances/electrical therapy skills station, case simulations, and core case tests. For a complete explanation of this algorithm, see the Recognition and Management of Cardiac Arrest chapter in the Provider Manual.

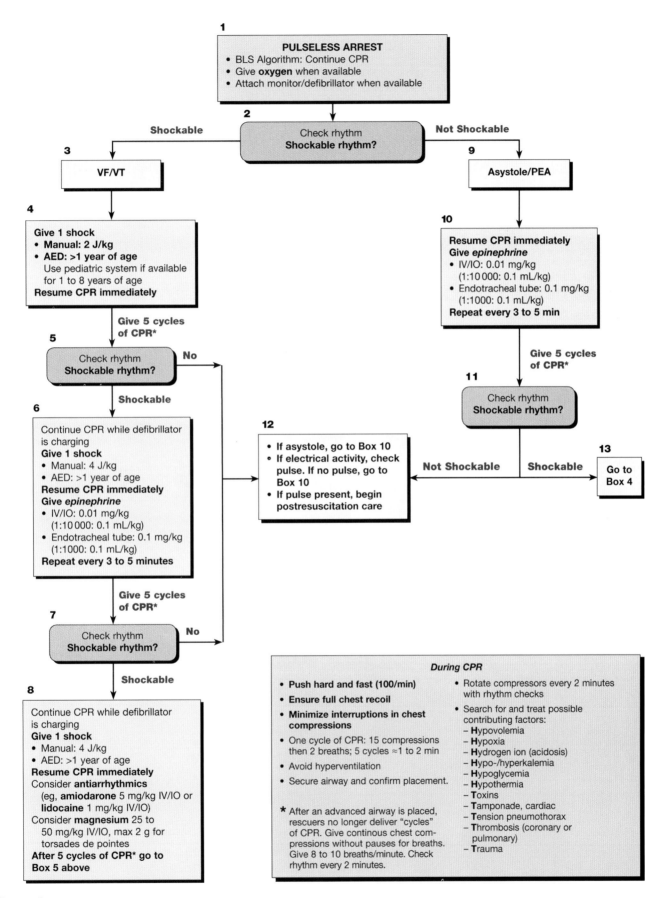

Figure 9. PALS Pulseless Arrest Algorithm.

Treatment Sequences for Cardiac Arrest

Introduction

Figures 10 and 11 illustrate the treatment sequences for cardiac arrest. Think of your management as a nearly continuous stream of CPR with minimal interruptions.

VF/Pulseless VT Treatment Sequence

Prepare next drug prior to rhythm check. Administer drug during CPR, as soon as possible after the rhythm check confirms VF/pulseless VT. Do not delay shock. Continue CPR while drugs are prepared and administered and defibrillator is charging. Ideally, chest compressions should be interrupted only for ventilation (until advanced airway placed), rhythm check, and actual shock delivery.

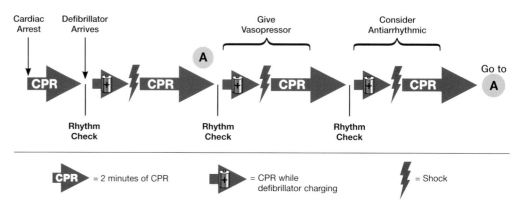

Figure 10. Pulseless arrest treatment sequences: ventricular fibrillation/pulseless ventricular tachycardia.

Asystole/PEA Treatment Sequence

Prepare next drug prior to rhythm check. Administer drug during CPR, as soon as possible after the rhythm check confirms no VF/pulseless VT. Continue CPR while drugs are prepared and administered. Ideally, chest compressions should be interrupted only for ventilation (until advanced airway placed) and rhythm check. Search for and treat possible contributing factors.

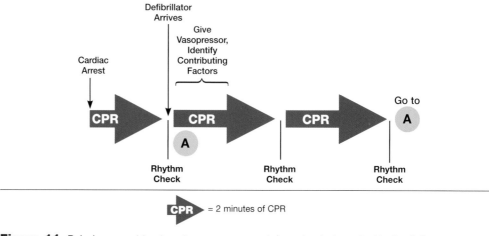

Figure 11. Pulseless arrest treatment sequences: asystole and pulseless electrical activity.

Length-Based/Color-Coded Resuscitation Tape

Summary

You should be familiar with using a reference for pediatric resuscitation drug doses and supplies, ie, a length-based/color-coded resuscitation tape (Figure 12). This tape gives an estimate of body weight based on a child's crown-to-heel length. In general practice drug doses for infants and children are based on body weight. In some emergency situations (eg, CPR), you can't weigh the critically ill or injured child and must estimate body weight. A length-based/color-coded resuscitation tape can be used to estimate body weight and to determine appropriate sizes of resuscitation supplies for a patient. The sizes of pediatric resuscitation supplies are organized and listed according to a color-coded length-based classification scheme.

Equipment	PINK Newborn/ Small infant (3-5 kg)	RED Infant (6-9 kg)	PURPLE Toddler (10-11 kg)	YELLOW Small Child (12-14 kg)	WHITE Child (15-18 kg)	BLUE Child (19-22 kg)	ORANGE Large Child (24-28 kg)	GREEN Adult (30-36 kg)
Resuscitation bag	Child	Child	Child	Child	Child	Child	Child/adult	Adult
O₂ mask	Newborn	Newborn	Pediatric	Pediatric	Pediatric	Pediatric	Adult	Adult
Oral airway	Infant/small child	Infant/small child	Small child	Child	Child	Child/small adult	Child/small adult	Medium adult
Laryngoscope blade (size)	0-1 straight	1 straight	1 straight	2 straight	2 straight or curved	2 straight or curved	2-3 straight or curved	3 straight or curved
Tracheal tube (mm)	Premature infant 2.5 Term infant 3.0-3.5 uncuffed	3.5 uncuffed	4.0 uncuffed	4.5 uncuffed	5.0 uncuffed	5.5 uncuffed	6.0 cuffed	6.5 cuffed
Endotracheal tube length (cm at lip)	10-10.5	10-10.5	11-12	12.5-13.5	14-15	15.5-16.5	17-18	18.5-19.5
Stylet (F)	6	6	6	6	6	14	14	14
Suction catheter (F)	6-8	8	8-10	10	10	10	10	12
BP cuff	Newborn/infant	Newborn/infant	Infant/child	Child	Child	Child	Child/adult	Adult
IV catheter (G)	22-24	22-24	20-24	18-22	18-22	18-20	18-20	16-20
Butterfly (G)	23-25	23-25	23-25	21-23	21-23	21-23	21-22	18-21
Nasogastric tube (F)	5-8	5-8	8-10	10	10-12	12-14	14-18	18
Urinary catheter (F)	5-8	5-8	8-10	10	10-12	10-12	12	12
Defibrillation/ cardioversion external paddles	Infant paddles	Infant paddles until 1 yr or 10 kg	Adult paddles when ≥1 yr or ≥10 kg	Adult paddles	Adult paddles	Adult paddles	Adult paddles	Adult paddles
Chest tube (F)	10-12	10-12	16-20	20-24	20-24	24-32	28-32	32-40

Figure 12. Pediatric resuscitation supplies based on color-coded resuscitation tape. Adapted from the 2002 Broselow Pediatric Resuscitation Tape, with permission from Armstrong Medical Industries, Lincolnshire, Ill. Modified from Hazinski MF, ed. *Manual of Pediatric Critical Care.* St. Louis, Mo: Mosby–Year Book; 1999.

Drugs Used in Cardiac Arrest

Summary

The following drugs may be used in cardiac arrest:

- Epinephrine
- Amiodarone HCl
- Lidocaine
- Magnesium sulfate
- Calcium chloride
- Atropine sulfate
- Sodium bicarbonate

See Part 10: Pharmacology for dosing and indications.

Cardiac Learning Station Competency Checklists 1-2

Cardiac Core Case 1 VF/Pulseless VT	Use this checklist during the PALS core case simulations and tests to check off the performance of the team leader.
Critical Performance Steps	**Details**
Team Leader	
___ **Assigns team member roles**	Team leader identifies self and assigns team roles
___ **Uses effective communication throughout**	Closed-loop communication Clear messages Clear roles and responsibilities Knowing one's limitations Knowledge sharing Constructive intervention Reevaluation and summarizing Mutual respect
Patient Management	
___ **Recognizes cardiopulmonary arrest**	Team leader directs or performs assessment to determine absence of responsiveness, breathing, and pulse
___ **Directs initiation of CPR and ensures performance of high-quality CPR at all times**	Team leader monitors quality of CPR (eg, presence of pulses with compressions, adequate rate, adequate depth, and chest recoil) and provides feedback to team member providing compressions; directs resuscitation so as to minimize interruptions in CPR; directs that team members rotate role of chest compressor approximately every 2 minutes
___ **Directs placement of pads/leads and activation of monitor**	Team leader directs that the pads/leads be properly placed and that the monitor be turned on to an appropriate lead
___ **Recognizes VF or pulseless VT**	Team leader recognizes rhythm and verbalizes presence of VF/VT to team members
___ **Directs attempted defibrillation at 2 J/kg safely**	Team leader directs team member to set proper energy and attempt defibrillation; observes for safe performance
___ **Directs immediate resumption of CPR**	Team leader directs team member to resume CPR immediately after shock (no pulse or rhythm check)
___ **Directs IV or IO access**	Team leader directs team member to place IO (or IV) line; line placement simulated properly
___ **Directs preparation of appropriate dose of epinephrine**	Team leader directs team member to prepare initial dose of epinephrine (0.01 mg/kg or 0.1 mL/kg of 1:10 000 IV/IO); uses drug dosing guide if needed

Cardiac Core Case 1 **VF/Pulseless VT** (continued)	
Critical Performance Steps	**Details**
___ **Directs attempted defibrillation at 4 J/kg safely**	Team leader tells team member to set proper energy and attempt defibrillation; observes for safe performance
___ **Directs immediate resumption of CPR**	Team leader directs team member to resume CPR immediately after shock (no pulse or rhythm check)
___ **Directs administration of epinephrine**	Team leader directs team member to administer epinephrine dose followed by saline flush
Case Conclusion	
___ **Verbalizes consideration of antiarrhythmic (amiodarone or lidocaine)**	Team leader indicates consideration of appropriate antiarrhythmic in proper dose

Cardiac Core Case 2 PEA/Asystole	Use this checklist during the PALS core case simulations and tests to check off the performance of the team leader.
Critical Performance Steps	**Details**
Team Leader	
___ **Assigns team member roles**	Team leader identifies self and assigns team roles
___ **Uses effective communication throughout**	Closed-loop communication Clear messages Clear roles and responsibilities Knowing one's limitations Knowledge sharing Constructive intervention Reevaluation and summarizing Mutual respect
Patient Management	
___ **Recognizes cardiopulmonary arrest**	Team leader directs or performs assessment to determine absence of responsiveness, breathing, and pulse
___ **Directs initiation of CPR and ensures performance of high-quality CPR at all times**	Team leader monitors quality of CPR (eg, adequate rate, adequate depth, and chest recoil) and provides feedback to team member providing compressions; directs resuscitation so as to minimize interruptions in CPR; directs that team members rotate role of chest compressor approximately every 2 minutes
___ **Directs placement of pads/leads and activation of monitor**	Team leader directs that pads/leads be properly placed and that the monitor be turned on to an appropriate lead
___ **Recognizes asystole or PEA**	Team leader recognizes rhythm and verbalizes presence of asystole or PEA to team members
___ **Directs IV or IO access**	Team leader directs team member to place IO (or IV) line; line placement simulated properly
___ **Directs preparation of appropriate dose of epinephrine**	Team leader directs team member to prepare initial dose of epinephrine (0.01 mg/kg or 0.1 mL/kg of 1:10 000 IV/IO), using drug resource if needed
___ **Directs administration of epinephrine at appropriate intervals**	Team leader directs team member to administer epinephrine dose with saline flush and prepare to administer again every 3 to 5 minutes
___ **Directs checking rhythm on the monitor approximately every 2 minutes**	Team leader directs team members to stop compressions and checks rhythm on monitor approximately every 2 minutes
Case Conclusion	
___ **Verbalizes consideration of at least 3 reversible causes of PEA or asystole**	Team leader verbalizes at least 3 potentially reversible causes of PEA or asystole (eg, hypovolemia, tamponade)

Part 7

Bradyarrhythmias and Tachyarrhythmias

Classification of Arrhythmias

Introduction

Cardiac rhythm disturbances (arrhythmias) occur as a result of abnormalities in the pacemaker or electrical conduction systems of the heart. They can also result from injury to the heart (eg, trauma, ischemia). An arrhythmia in a child can be broadly classified as follows:

Heart Rate	Classification
Slow	Bradyarrhythmia
Fast	Tachyarrhythmia
Absent	Pulseless arrest

This part reviews the recognition and management of arrhythmias with pulses. Part 6: Cardiac Arrest discusses pulseless arrest.

Bradyarrhythmias

Definition

Bradycardia is defined as a heart rate that is slow compared with normal heart rates for patient age (Table 3). A relative bradycardia is defined as a heart rate that is too low for the child's level of activity and clinical condition.

Table 3. Heart Rate in Children

Heart Rate (bpm)* Age	Awake Rate	Mean	Sleeping Rate
Newborn to 3 months	85 to 205	140	80 to 160
3 months to 2 years	100 to 190	130	75 to 160
2 to 10 years	60 to 140	80	60 to 90
>10 years	60 to 100	75	50 to 90

Signs of Bradyarrhythmias

Bradyarrhythmias may present with nonspecific symptoms, such as lightheadedness, dizziness, syncope, and fatigue. The cardinal signs of instability associated with bradyarrhythmias are

- shock with hypotension
- poor end-organ perfusion
- altered level of consciousness, sometimes with slow or absent ventilation
- sudden collapse

The rhythm is unstable if it is producing significant symptoms, and it may deteriorate to cardiac arrest.

Symptomatic bradycardia requiring urgent treatment is defined as a heart rate slower than normal for patient age associated with evidence of shock (eg, poor systemic perfusion, hypotension, altered consciousness) and/or respiratory distress or failure.

Tachyarrhythmias

Definition

Tachycardia is defined as a heart rate that is fast compared with normal heart rates for the patient's age (Table 3). A relative tachycardia is a heart rate that is too fast for the child's level of activity and clinical condition.

Signs of Tachyarrhythmias

Tachyarrhythmias may present with nonspecific symptoms that vary according to the age of the patient. Symptoms may include lightheadedness, dizziness, fatigue, and syncope. Infants may be irritable or lethargic. Episodes of extremely rapid heart rate can be life-threatening.

The cardinal signs of instability associated with tachyarrhythmias are

- respiratory distress/failure
- shock with hypotension
- poor end-organ perfusion
- altered level of consciousness
- sudden collapse

The rhythm is unstable if it produces significant symptoms, and it may deteriorate to cardiac arrest.

Classification of Tachyarrhythmias

Tachyarrhythmias may be generally classified according to the width of the QRS complex, either narrow complex or wide complex:

Narrow Complex	Wide Complex
• Sinus tachycardia	• Supraventricular tachycardia (with aberrant conduction)
• Atrial flutter	• Ventricular tachycardia
• Supraventricular tachycardia (SVT)	

Resources

Read the Recognition and Management of Bradyarrhythmias and Tachyarrhythmias chapter in the Provider Manual for more information.

Rhythm Strips: Bradyarrhythmias and Tachyarrhythmias

Introduction

You must be able to identify bradyarrhythmias (ie, sinus bradycardia) and tachyarrhythmias (ie, sinus tachycardia, SVT, and VT) throughout the course. Study the following rhythm strips to prepare for the rhythm disturbances/electrical therapy skills stations, the case simulations, and the core case tests.

Bradyarrhythmias

Sinus Bradycardia

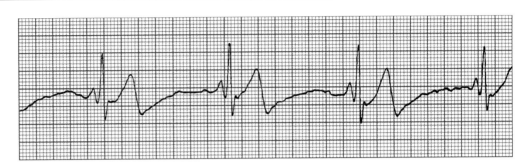

Figure 13. Sinus bradycardia.

Narrow-Complex Tachyarrhythmias

Sinus Tachycardia

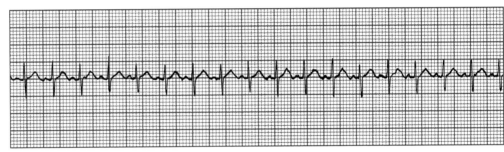

Figure 14. Sinus tachycardia.

SVT

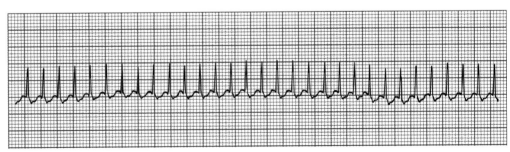

Figure 15. Supraventricular tachycardia (SVT).

SVT Converting to Sinus Rhythm

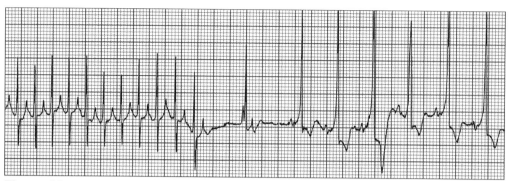

Figure 16. SVT converting to sinus rhythm with adenosine administration.

Wide-Complex Tachyarrhythmia

Ventricular Tachycardia (Monomorphic)

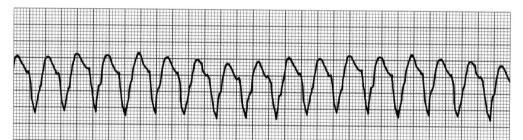

Figure 17. Ventricular tachycardia (monomorphic).

PALS Bradycardia With a Pulse Algorithm

Introduction

Study the PALS Bradycardia With a Pulse Algorithm (Figure 18) to prepare for the course. You will be presented with symptomatic bradycardia scenarios during the rhythm disturbances/electrical therapy skills station, case simulations, and PALS core case tests. For a complete explanation of this algorithm, see the Recognition and Management of Bradyarrhythmias and Tachyarrhythmias chapter in the Provider Manual.

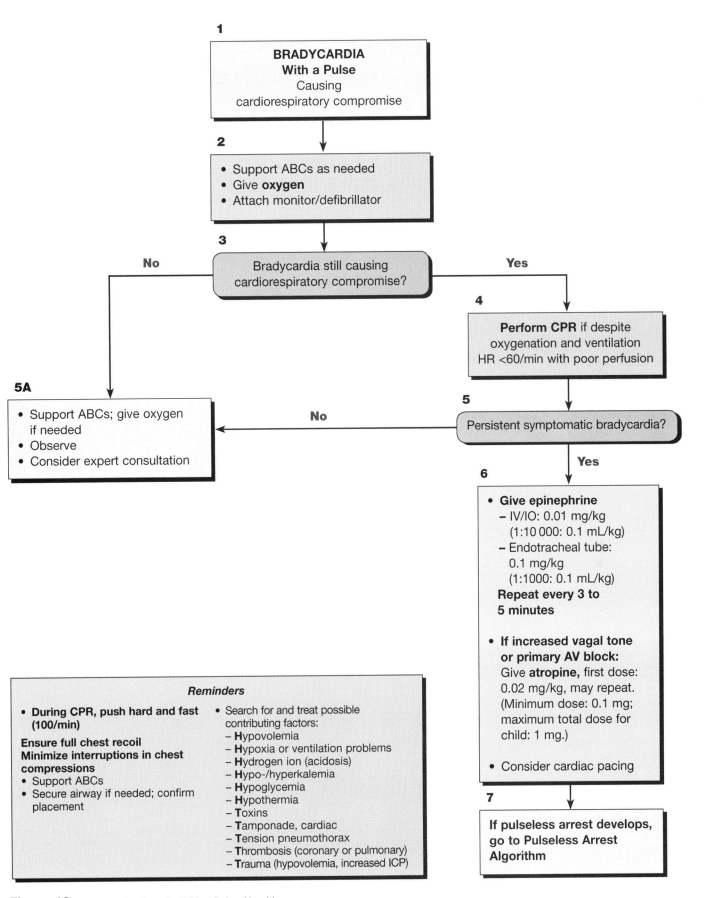

1
BRADYCARDIA
With a Pulse
Causing
cardiorespiratory compromise

2
- Support ABCs as needed
- Give **oxygen**
- Attach monitor/defibrillator

3
Bradycardia still causing cardiorespiratory compromise?

No

Yes

4
Perform CPR if despite oxygenation and ventilation HR <60/min with poor perfusion

5A
- Support ABCs; give oxygen if needed
- Observe
- Consider expert consultation

No

5
Persistent symptomatic bradycardia?

Yes

6
- **Give epinephrine**
  - IV/IO: 0.01 mg/kg (1:10 000: 0.1 mL/kg)
  - Endotracheal tube: 0.1 mg/kg (1:1000: 0.1 mL/kg)
  Repeat every 3 to 5 minutes

- **If increased vagal tone or primary AV block:** Give **atropine,** first dose: 0.02 mg/kg, may repeat. (Minimum dose: 0.1 mg; maximum total dose for child: 1 mg.)

- Consider cardiac pacing

7
If pulseless arrest develops, go to Pulseless Arrest Algorithm

Reminders

- **During CPR, push hard and fast (100/min)**

Ensure full chest recoil
Minimize interruptions in chest compressions
- Support ABCs
- Secure airway if needed; confirm placement

- Search for and treat possible contributing factors:
  - **H**ypovolemia
  - **H**ypoxia or ventilation problems
  - **H**ydrogen ion (acidosis)
  - **H**ypo-/hyperkalemia
  - **H**ypoglycemia
  - **H**ypothermia
  - **T**oxins
  - **T**amponade, cardiac
  - **T**ension pneumothorax
  - **T**hrombosis (coronary or pulmonary)
  - **T**rauma (hypovolemia, increased ICP)

Figure 18. Pediatric Bradycardia With a Pulse Algorithm.

PALS Tachycardia With Pulses and Poor Perfusion Algorithm

Introduction

Study the PALS Tachycardia With Pulses and Poor Perfusion Algorithm (Figure 19) to prepare for the course. You will be presented with symptomatic tachycardia scenarios during the rhythm disturbances/electrical therapy skills station, case simulations, and core case tests. For a complete explanation of this algorithm, see the Recognition and Management of Bradyarrhythmias and Tachyarrhythmias chapter in the Provider Manual.

Drugs for Bradyarrhythmias and Tachyarrhythmias

Summary

Drugs that may be used to treat bradyarrhythmias are

- atropine
- epinephrine

Drugs that may be used to treat tachyarrhythmias are

- adenosine
- amiodarone
- lidocaine
- procainamide
- sodium bicarbonate

See Part 10: Pharmacology for dosing and indications.

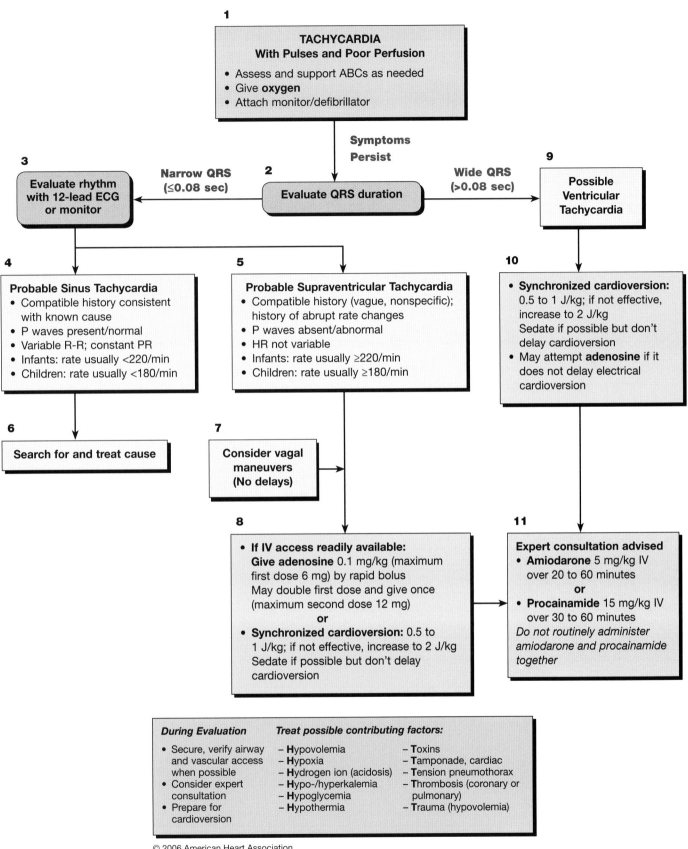

Figure 19. Pediatric Tachycardia With Pulses and Poor Perfusion Algorithm.

Cardiac Learning Station Competency Checklists 3-4

Cardiac Core Case 3 Tachycardia (SVT)	Use this checklist during the PALS core case simulations and tests to check off the performance of the team leader.
Critical Performance Steps	**Details**
Team Leader	
___ **Assigns team member roles**	Team leader identifies self and assigns team roles
___ **Uses effective communication throughout**	Closed-loop communication Clear messages Clear roles and responsibilities Knowing one's limitations Knowledge sharing Constructive intervention Reevaluation and summarizing Mutual respect
Patient Management	
___ **Directs assessment of airway, breathing, circulation, disability, and exposure, including vital signs**	Team leader directs or performs assessment to determine airway patency, adequacy of breathing and circulation, level of responsiveness, temperature, and vital signs
___ **Directs administration of supplemental oxygen**	Team leader directs administration of supplementary oxygen by high-flow device
___ **Directs placement of pads/leads and pulse oximetry**	Team leader directs that pads/leads be properly placed and that the monitor be turned on to an appropriate lead and requests use of pulse oximetry
___ **Recognizes narrow-complex tachycardia and verbalizes how to distinguish between ST and SVT**	Team leader recognizes narrow-complex tachycardia and verbalizes reasons for identification as SVT vs ST
___ **Categorizes as compensated or hypotensive**	Team leader verbalizes whether patient is compensated or hypotensive
___ **Directs performance of appropriate vagal maneuvers**	Team leader directs team member to perform appropriate vagal maneuvers (eg, Valsalva, blowing through straw, ice to face)
___ **Directs IV or IO access**	Team leader directs team member to place IO (or IV) line; line placement simulated properly
___ **Directs preparation and administration of appropriate dose of adenosine**	Team leader directs team member to prepare correct dose of adenosine; uses drug dose resource if needed. States need for rapid administration with use of saline flush
___ **Directs reassessment of patient in response to treatment**	Team leader directs team member to reassess airway, breathing, and circulation

Cardiac Core Case 3 Tachycardia (SVT)	*Use this checklist during the PALS core case simulations and tests to check off the performance of the team leader.*
Critical Performance Steps	**Details**
Case Conclusion	
___ **Verbalizes indications and appropriate energy doses for synchronized cardioversion**	Team leader verbalizes indications and correct energy dose for synchronized cardioversion (0.5 to 1 J/kg)

Cardiac Core Case 4 Bradycardia	Use this checklist during the PALS core case simulations and tests to check off the performance of the team leader.
Critical Performance Steps	**Details**
Team Leader	
____ **Assigns team member roles**	Team leader identifies self and assigns team roles
____ **Uses effective communication throughout**	Closed-loop communication Clear messages Clear roles and responsibilities Knowing one's limitations Knowledge sharing Constructive intervention Reevaluation and summarizing Mutual respect
Patient Managment	
____ **Directs assessment of airway, breathing, circulation, disability, and exposure, including vital signs**	Team leader directs or performs assessment to determine airway patency, adequacy of breathing and circulation, level of responsiveness, temperature, and vital signs
____ **Directs initiation of assisted ventilations with 100% oxygen**	Team leader instructs team member to provide assisted ventilations with 100% oxygen
____ **Directs placement of pads/leads and activation of monitor and requests pulse oximetry**	Team leader directs that pads/leads be properly placed and that monitor be turned on to an appropriate lead; requests use of pulse oximetry
____ **Recognizes bradycardia with cardiorespiratory compromise**	Team leader recognizes rhythm and verbalizes presence of bradycardia to team members
____ **Characterizes as compensated or hypotensive**	Team leader communicates that patient has cardiorespiratory compromise and is hypotensive
____ **Recalls indications for chest compressions in a bradycardic patient**	Team leader verbalizes indications for chest compressions (may or may not perform)
____ **Directs IV or IO access**	Team leader directs team member to place IO (or IV) line; line placement simulated properly
____ **Directs preparation and administration of appropriate dose of epinephrine**	Team leader directs team member to prepare initial dose of epinephrine; uses drug dose resource if needed; directs team member to administer epinephrine dose and saline flush
____ **Directs reassessment of patient in response to treatment**	Team leader directs team members to reassess airway, breathing, and circulation
Case Conclusion	
____ **Verbalizes consideration of at least 3 underlying causes of bradycardia**	Team leader verbalizes potentially reversible causes of bradycardia (eg, toxins, hypothermia, increased ICP)

Part 8

Respiratory Emergencies

Categorization of Respiratory Problem by Severity

Introduction

It is typically not difficult to distinguish a child who is breathing from one who is not. But it can be difficult to distinguish on clinical grounds a child who is merely working hard to breathe (in respiratory distress) from one who is in severe distress and deteriorating toward full respiratory arrest (in respiratory failure). You must be alert to respiratory conditions that are treatable with simple measures (eg, administration of oxygen or nebulized albuterol). It may be even more important to identify respiratory conditions that are subtly, yet rapidly, progressing toward cardiopulmonary failure. These conditions require timely intervention with support of airway and ventilation (eg, assisted bag-mask ventilation).

The earlier you detect and treat respiratory distress and respiratory failure, the better chance the child has for a good outcome.

Definition of Respiratory Distress

Respiratory distress is a clinical state characterized by increased respiratory rate (tachypnea) and increased respiratory effort (resulting in nasal flaring, retractions, and use of accessory muscles). Respiratory distress can be associated with changes in airway sounds, skin color, and mental status.

Definition of Respiratory Failure

Respiratory failure is a clinical state of inadequate oxygenation, ventilation, or both. It may be characterized by signs of respiratory distress or inadequate respiratory effort. Diagnosis of respiratory failure may require laboratory testing (eg, arterial blood gas).

Categorization of Respiratory Problem by Type

Types of Respiratory Illness

Respiratory problems can be classified into one or more of the following types:

- Upper airway obstruction
- Lower airway obstruction
- Lung tissue (parenchymal) disease
- Disordered control of breathing

Respiratory problems do not always occur in isolation. Any or all types may be present at the same time. For example, a child may present with status asthmaticus (lower airway obstruction) and viral pneumonitis (lung tissue disease). Another child may have bronchospasm (lower airway obstruction) and respiratory muscle weakness (disordered control of breathing) due to organophosphate poisoning.

P a r t 8

Resources

See the Recognition of Respiratory Distress and Failure chapter and the Management of Respiratory Distress and Failure chapter in the Provider Manual for a complete discussion.

Use of the Pediatric Assessment Approach in Evaluating Respiratory Problems

Introduction

Use the systematic approach to pediatric assessment when evaluating a seriously ill or injured child with a respiratory problem.

General Assessment

Look and listen for the following signs of respiratory distress or failure in the initial quick visual and auditory evaluation of the child:

Appearance—Appearance will vary depending on the severity of the respiratory condition. A child with mild respiratory distress may be compensating and may have tachypnea but otherwise appear normal. A child with more severe disease may be alert and interactive but anxious. A child in respiratory failure may appear very ill and have tachypnea, sweating, half-closed eyelids, and a look that says "Help me!" A child with respiratory symptoms who is lethargic or unresponsive is very worrisome and suggests respiratory failure and possible imminent respiratory arrest.

Work of breathing—The child may have an increased respiratory rate, increased respiratory effort, and abnormal airway and audible lung sounds (eg, grunting, wheezing). Head bobbing or seesawing respirations are signs of severe distress and may precede rapid deterioration. As you observe the child, note whether breathing difficulty is seen during the inspiratory or expiratory phase. A child with increased respiratory effort may have difficulty speaking more than a few words at a time. An infant with increased respiratory effort may have a weak cry.

Circulation—The child may have normal or pale skin or frank cyanosis. Normal skin color is *not* necessarily a reliable sign of adequate oxygenation or ventilation. Cyanosis, particularly of the oral mucous membranes, indicates severe hypoxemia. Visible cyanosis, however, requires an adequate concentration of hemoglobin, so it may not be observed in an anemic child with hypoxemia. The child needs immediate high concentration of oxygen and possibly assisted ventilation.

Primary Assessment

If you suspect respiratory distress or respiratory failure, evaluate the child using the primary assessment. Pay particular attention to the signs discussed below.

> *If you observe a life-threatening condition (ie, imminent respiratory arrest associated with severe increase in work of breathing, slowing of respiratory rate associated with deteriorating level of consciousness) be prepared to support the airway, oxygenation, and ventilation.*

Airway

Evaluate the airway for airway compromise. Determine if the airway is clear or obstructed. If the upper airway is obstructed, you may observe

- increased inspiratory effort with retractions
- inspiratory sounds (snoring or high-pitched sounds [stridor])
- episodes of no airway sounds despite respiratory effort (ie, severe upper airway obstruction)
- inability to make any sounds (severe airway obstruction)
- copious nasal or oral secretions

If you identify a mild or severe airway obstruction, determine if you can maintain airway patency with simple measures, such as positioning and suctioning, or if advanced interventions are required.

Breathing

Evaluate breathing for findings of ventilatory compromise (ie, respiratory distress, respiratory failure, or imminent respiratory arrest).

Ventilatory Compromise

Signs of ventilatory compromise include the following:

- Unequal or absent breath sounds
- Asymmetric, diminished, paradoxical, or absent chest expansion during inspiration
  - Decreased chest expansion may result from conditions such as inadequate effort, airway obstruction, atelectasis, pneumothorax, hemothorax, pleural effusion, mucous plug, or foreign-body aspiration
  - Paradoxical chest movement is seen with upper airway obstruction and respiratory muscle weakness
- Diminished distal air entry—barely audible breath sounds auscultated distally
  - Decreased chest excursion with decreased air movement on lung auscultation often accompanies poor respiratory effort
  - Increased respiratory effort, chest excursion, and retractions combined with diminished distal air entry suggest airflow obstruction or lung tissue disease

Respiratory Distress

Evaluate for signs of respiratory distress:

Tachypnea	Tachypnea is often the first sign of respiratory distress, particularly in infants.
Increased respiratory effort (retractions, nasal flaring)	Retractions accompanied by inspiratory stridor or snoring sounds suggest upper airway obstruction. Retractions accompanied by expiratory wheezing suggest lower airway obstruction. Retractions accompanied by grunting and a rapid respiratory rate suggest lung tissue disease.
Grunting	Grunting is often a sign of lung tissue disease resulting from small airway collapse, alveolar collapse, or both. Respiratory conditions that cause grunting include pneumonia, acute respiratory distress syndrome, pulmonary contusion, and congestive heart failure causing pulmonary edema. Grunting may indicate progression of respiratory distress to respiratory failure.
Stridor	Stridor is typically a sign of extrathoracic upper airway obstruction (heard on inspiration). In rare cases it can be a sign of localized intrathoracic lower airway obstruction (heard on expiration). Causes of inspiratory stridor include foreign-body aspiration, congenital airway abnormality (eg, large tongue or laryngeal web), acquired airway abnormality (eg, tumor or cyst), infection (eg, croup), or upper airway edema (eg, allergic reaction or subglottic edema from ET tube trauma).
Wheezing	Wheezing is a sign of intrathoracic lower airway obstruction. Common causes of wheezing include bronchiolitis and asthma. Wheezing is most prominent during expiration. Inspiratory wheezing suggests a foreign body or other cause of obstruction in the trachea or upper airway. Inspiratory combined with expiratory wheezing also may be observed in severe asthma.
Seesawing or "abdominal" breathing	Abdominal breathing, a breathing pattern of severe chest retractions during inspiration accompanied by expansion of the abdomen, indicates extreme increase in work of breathing. It is often a sign of upper airway obstruction. It is also commonly seen in children with neuromuscular weakness. This inefficient form of ventilation may quickly lead to fatigue and progression to respiratory failure.
Head bobbing	Head bobbing, a sign of markedly increased respiratory effort, may be observed in respiratory failure, particularly in newborns and young infants.

Imminent Respiratory Arrest

Evaluate for signs of imminent respiratory arrest, such as

- bradypnea
- periodic apnea
- falling heart rate/bradycardia
- diminished air movement
- low oxyhemoglobin saturation
- stupor, coma
- poor skeletal muscle tone
- cyanosis

Always evaluate changes in respiratory rate in light of other clinical findings. A decrease in respiratory rate from a rapid to a more "normal" rate may indicate improvement if accompanied by improved mental status and reduced signs of air hunger. But a decreasing or irregular respiratory rate in a child with a deteriorating level of consciousness typically indicates worsening respiratory disease.

Circulation

Evaluate for evidence of coexisting shock. Respiratory problems may produce cardiovascular changes, including compromise in cardiovascular and end-organ perfusion and function. Respiratory failure with extreme reduction in oxygen delivery or acidosis can impair stroke volume (ie, the amount of blood pumped with each heartbeat), heart rate, and cardiac output. Evaluate cardiovascular function, including heart rate, rhythm, and systemic perfusion, to detect signs of cardiovascular compromise in every child exhibiting respiratory distress or failure.

One of the earliest cardiovascular changes in a child in respiratory distress or failure is tachycardia. This rapid heart rate is a response to the stress, pain, fever, hypoxia, hypercarbia, or other factors associated with the illness. Bradycardia is often a sign of hypoxia and may indicate that respiratory arrest is imminent.

Cardiovascular Function Compromise

Look for these signs of cardiovascular function compromise (ie, shock):

- Tachycardia
- Bradycardia
- Diminished peripheral pulses
- Diminished central pulses (imminent arrest)
- Abnormal capillary refill
- Hypotension

End-Organ Function Compromise

Look for these signs of end-organ function compromise:

- Cool, pale, diaphoretic skin, cyanosis
- Decreased urine output
- Changes in mental status (see next section)

Disability

Evaluate for changes in mental status and pupillary responses. Signs of deterioration in neurologic function are changes in eye opening, verbal responses, and motor function, including decreased muscle tone.

Mental Status	Evaluation of mental status is an integral part of the disability assessment. Altered mental status is a critical indicator of both inadequate oxygenation and inadequate ventilation. It can also indicate inadequate cerebral perfusion or an abnormal metabolic state affecting brain function. A child with a decreased level of consciousness caused by impaired oxygenation needs supplementary oxygen. The same child, however, may also be suffering from inadequate ventilation. Because oxyhemoglobin saturation indicated by pulse oximetry may be normal after supplementary oxygen is administered, the inadequate ventilation may go undiagnosed.

Pupillary Responses	Pupillary responses are preserved in metabolic states such as hypoxia due to respiratory illness. Enlarged pupils can be evidence of sympathetic stimulation induced by hypoxemia or hypercarbia, but they will remain reactive.

Exposure	Evaluate by exposing the child for a complete physical examination. Assess core temperature and avoid exposure hypothermia. Exposure provides important information leading to the diagnosis of the underlying respiratory condition and allows for • direct observation of the chest wall and mechanics of breathing • observation of adequacy and symmetry of chest rise • assessment of intercostal and sternal retractions

Recognition of Respiratory Problems Flowchart

Introduction	Figure 20 outlines the approach to recognizing the type and severity of a respiratory problem. At any point during your evaluation, be alert to life-threatening conditions. If you identify one, intervene immediately and activate the ERS.

Pediatric Advanced Life Support
Recognition of Respiratory Problems

Clinical Signs		Upper Airway Obstruction	Lower Airway Obstruction	Lung Tissue (Parenchymal) Disease	Disordered Control of Breathing
A	Patency	Airway open and maintainable/not maintainable			
B	Respiratory rate/effort	Increased			Variable
B	Breath Sounds	Stridor (typically inspiratory) Seal-like cough Hoarseness	Wheezing (typically expiratory) Prolonged expiratory phase	Grunting Crackles Decreased breath sounds	Normal
B	Air Movement	Decreased			Variable
C	Heart Rate	Tachycardia (early) Bradycardia (late)			
C	Skin	Pallor, cool skin (early) Cyanosis (late)			
D	Level of Consciousness	Anxiety, agitation (early) Lethargy, unresponsiveness (late)			
E	Temperature	Variable			

Pediatric Advanced Life Support
Categorize Respiratory Problems by Severity

Respiratory Distress → **Respiratory Failure**

A — Open and maintainable → **Not maintainable**

B — Tachypnea → **Bradypnea to apnea**

Work of breathing (nasal flaring/retractions)
Increased effort → **Decreased effort** → **Apnea**

Good air movement → **Poor to absent air movement**

C — Tachycardia → **Bradycardia**

Pallor → **Cyanosis**

D — Anxiety, agitation → **Lethargy to unresponsiveness**

E — Variable temperature

Figure 20. Recognition of Respiratory Problems Flowchart

Fundamentals of Respiratory Management

Management of Respiratory Emergencies Flowchart

Figure 21 outlines general management of respiratory emergencies and specific management according to the type of respiratory problem. Please note that this chart does not include all respiratory emergencies; it provides key management strategies for a limited number of diseases.

Management of Respiratory Emergencies Flowchart

- Airway positioning
- Oxygen
- Pulse oximetry
- ECG monitor (as indicated)
- BLS as indicated

Upper Airway Obstruction
Specific Management for Selected Conditions

Croup	Anaphylaxis	Aspiration Foreign Body
• Nebulized epinephrine • Corticosteroids	• IM epinephrine (or auto-injector) • Albuterol • Antihistamines • Corticosteroids	• Allow position of comfort • Specialty consultation

Lower Airway Obstruction
Specific Management for Selected Conditions

Bronchiolitis	Asthma
• Nasal suctioning • Bronchodilator trial	• Albuterol ± ipratropium • Corticosteroids • SQ epinephrine • Magnesium sulfate • Terbutaline

Lung Tissue (Parenchymal) Disease
Specific Management for Selected Conditions

Pneumonia/Pneumonitis *Infectious Chemical Aspiration*	Pulmonary Edema *Cardiogenic or Noncardiogenic (ARDS)*
• Albuterol • Antibiotics (as indicated)	• Consider noninvasive or invasive ventilatory support with PEEP • Consider vasoactive support • Consider diuretic

Disordered Control of Breathing
Specific Management for Selected Conditions

Increased ICP	Poisoning/Overdose	Neuromuscular Disease
• Avoid hypoxemia • Avoid hypercarbia • Avoid hyperthermia	• Antidote (if available) • Contact poison control	• Consider noninvasive or invasive ventilatory suport

Figure 21. Management of Respiratory Emergencies Flowchart

Drugs Used in Respiratory Emergencies

The following drugs may be used in the management of respiratory emergencies:

- Albuterol
- Corticosteroids (Dexamethasone, Methylprednisolone)
- Diphenhydramine
- Epinephrine (racemic or L-epinephrine)
- Furosemide
- Ipratropium bromide
- Magnesium sulfate
- Oxygen
- Terbutaline

See the Management of Respiratory Distress and Failure chapter in the Provider Manual and Part 10: Pharmacology for more information.

Respiratory Learning Station Competency Checklists 1-4

Introduction

The following pages are the learning station competency checklists for Respiratory Core Cases 1-4.

Respiratory Core Case 1 Upper Airway Obstruction	Use this checklist during the PALS core case simulations and tests to check off the performance of the team leader.
Critical Performance Steps	**Details**
Team Leader	
___ **Assigns team member roles**	Team leader identifies self and assigns team roles
___ **Uses effective communication throughout**	Closed-loop communication Clear messages Clear roles and responsibilities Knowing one's limitations Knowledge sharing Constructive intervention Reevaluation and summarizing Mutual respect
Patient Management	
___ **Directs assessment of airway, breathing, circulation, disability, and exposure, including vital signs**	Team leader directs or performs assessment to determine responsiveness, breathing, and pulse
___ **Directs manual airway maneuver with administration of 100% oxygen**	Directs manual airway maneuver and administration of 100% oxygen
___ **Directs placement of pads/leads and pulse oximetry**	Team leader directs that pads/leads be properly placed and that the monitor be turned on to an appropriate lead; requests use of pulse oximetry
___ **Recognizes signs and symptoms of upper airway obstruction**	Team leader verbalizes features of history and exam that indicate upper airway obstruction
___ **Categorizes as respiratory distress or failure**	Team leader verbalizes whether patient is in respiratory distress or failure
___ **Verbalizes indications for assisted ventilations or CPAP**	Team leader verbalizes that for patient with ineffective ventilations or poor oxygenation, assisted ventilations are required
___ **Directs IV or IO access**	Team leader directs team member to place IO (or IV); line placement simulated properly
___ **Directs reassessment of patient in response to treatment**	Team leader directs team member to reassess airway, breathing, and circulation
Case Conclusion	
___ **Summarizes specific treatments for upper airway obstruction**	Team leader summarizes specific treatments for upper airway obstruction (eg, racemic epinephrine, CPAP)
___ *If scope of practice applies:* **Verbalizes indications for endotracheal intubation and special considerations when intubation is anticipated**	*If scope of practice applies:* Verbalizes indications for endotracheal intubation (decreased mental status, inadequate oxygenation). Notes need to anticipate use of an ET tube smaller than predicted for age, especially if subglottic narrowing is suspected.

Respiratory Core Case 2 Lower Airway Obstruction	Use this checklist during the PALS core case simulations and tests to check off the performance of the team leader.
Critical Performance Steps	**Details**
Team Leader	
___ **Assigns team member roles**	Team leader identifies self and assigns team roles
___ **Uses effective communication throughout**	Closed-loop communication Clear messages Clear roles and responsibilities Knowing one's limitations Knowledge sharing Constructive intervention Reevaluation and summarizing Mutual respect
Patient Management	
___ **Directs assessment of airway, breathing, circulation, disability, and exposure, including vital signs**	Team leader directs or performs assessment to determine airway patency, adequacy of breathing and circulation, level of responsiveness, temperature, and vital signs
___ **Directs administration of 100% oxygen**	Team leader instructs team member to provide 100% oxygen
___ **Directs placement of pads/leads and pulse oximetry**	Team leader directs that pads/leads be properly placed and that the monitor be turned on to an appropriate lead; requests use of pulse oximetry
___ **Recognizes signs and symptoms of lower airway obstruction**	Team leader verbalizes features of history and exam that indicate lower airway obstruction
___ **Categorizes as respiratory distress or failure**	Team leader verbalizes whether patient has respiratory distress or failure
___ **Verbalizes indications for assisted ventilations**	Team leader verbalizes that for patient with ineffective ventilations or poor oxygenation, assisted ventilations are required
___ **Directs IV or IO access**	Team leader directs team member to place IO (or IV) line; line placement simulated properly
___ **Directs reassessment of patient in response to treatment**	Team leader directs team members to reassess airway, breathing, and circulation
Case Conclusion	
___ **Summarizes specific treatments for lower airway obstruction**	Team leader summarizes specific treatments for lower airway obstruction (eg, nebulized albuterol)
___ *If scope of practice applies:* **Verbalizes indications for endotracheal intubation**	*If scope of practice applies:* Verbalizes indications for endotracheal intubation (decreased mental status, inadequate oxygenation)

Respiratory Core Case 3 Lung Tissue (Parenchymal) Disease	Use this checklist during the PALS core case simulations and tests to check off the performance of the team leader.
Critical Performance Steps	**Details**
Team Leader	.
___ **Assigns team member roles**	Team leader identifies self and assigns team roles
___ **Uses effective communication throughout**	Closed-loop communication Clear messages Clear roles and responsibilities Knowing one's limitations Knowledge sharing Constructive intervention Reevaluation and summarizing Mutual respect
Patient Management	
___ **Directs assessment of airway, breathing, circulation, disability, and exposure, including vital signs**	Team leader directs or performs assessment to determine airway patency, adequacy of breathing and circulation, level of responsiveness, temperature, and vital signs
___ **Directs assisted ventilations with 100% oxygen**	Team leader directs initiation of assisted ventilations with 100% oxygen
___ **Ensures that bag-mask ventilations are effective**	Team leader observes or directs team member to observe for chest rise and breath sounds
___ **Directs placement of pads/leads and pulse oximetry**	Team leader directs that pads/leads be properly placed and that the monitor be turned on to an appropriate lead; requests use of pulse oximetry
___ **Recognizes signs and symptoms of lung tissue (parenchymal) disease**	Team leader verbalizes features of history and exam that indicate lung tissue (parenchymal) disease
___ **Categorizes as respiratory distress or failure**	Team leader verbalizes whether patient is in respiratory distress or failure
___ **Directs IV or IO access**	Team leader directs team member to place IO (or IV) line; line placement simulated properly
___ **Directs reassessment of patient in response to treatment**	Team leader directs team members to reassess airway, breathing, and circulation
Case Conclusion	
___ **Summarizes specific treatments for lung tissue (parenchymal) disease**	Team leader summarizes specific treatments for lung tissue (parenchymal) disease (eg, antibiotics for suspected pneumonia)
___ *If scope of practice applies:* **Verbalizes indications for endotracheal intubation**	*If scope of practice applies:* Verbalizes indications for endotracheal intubation (decreased mental status, inadequate oxygenation)

Respiratory Core Case 4 Disordered Control of Breathing	*Use this checklist during the PALS core case simulations and tests to check off the performance of the team leader.*
Critical Performance Steps	**Details**
Team Leader	
___ **Assigns team member roles**	Team leader identifies self and assigns team roles
___ **Uses effective communication throughout**	Closed-loop communication Clear messages Clear roles and responsibilities Knowing one's limitations Knowledge sharing Constructive intervention Reevaluation and summarizing Mutual respect
Patient Management	
___ **Directs assessment of airway, breathing, circulation, disability, and exposure, including vital signs**	Team leader directs or performs assessment to determine airway patency, adequacy of breathing and circulation, level of responsiveness, temperature, and vital signs
___ **Directs assisted ventilations with 100% oxygen**	Team leader directs assisted ventilations with 100% oxygen
___ **Ensures that bag-mask ventilations are effective**	Team leader ensures that there is chest rise with assisted ventilations
___ **Directs placement of pads/leads and pulse oximetry**	Team leader directs that pads/leads be properly placed and that the monitor be turned on to an appropriate lead; requests use of pulse oximetry
___ **Recognizes signs and symptoms of disordered control of breathing**	Team leader verbalizes features of history and exam that indicate disordered control of breathing
___ **Categorizes as respiratory distress or failure**	Team leader verbalizes whether patient is in respiratory distress or failure (note that respiratory failure can occur without distress in this setting)
___ **Directs IV or IO access**	Team leader directs team member to place IO (or IV) line; line placement simulated properly
___ **Directs reassessment of patient in response to treatment**	Team leader observes or directs other team members to reassess airway, breathing, and circulation
Case Conclusion	
___ **Summarizes specific treatments for disordered control of breathing**	Team leader summarizes specific treatments for disordered control of breathing (eg, reversal agents)
___ *If scope of practice applies:* **Verbalizes indications for endotracheal intubation**	*If scope of practice applies:* Verbalizes indications for endotracheal intubation (decreased mental status, inadequate respiratory effort or oxygenation)

Part 9

Shock

Categorization of Shock by Severity

Introduction

Outcomes in seriously ill or injured children can be greatly improved with *early recognition and treatment* of shock. If left untreated, shock can quickly progress to cardiopulmonary failure and cardiac arrest. Survival from cardiac arrest is poor.

The earlier you recognize shock, establish priorities, and start therapy, the better the child's chance for a good outcome.

Definition of Shock

Shock is a critical condition that results from inadequate delivery of oxygen and nutrients to the tissues to meet metabolic demand. Shock is often characterized by inadequate perfusion. In children most shock is characterized by low cardiac output.

Inadequate delivery of oxygen and removal of metabolites can lead to tissue hypoxia, anaerobic metabolism, accumulation of lactic acid and carbon dioxide, and irreversible cellular damage. Death may then rapidly result from cardiovascular collapse or later from multiple-organ system failure. Conditions such as fever, increased work of breathing, injury, agitation, and pain may contribute to shock by increasing tissue demand for oxygen and nutrients. Whether due to inadequate supply of oxygen to the tissues or increased demand of the tissues for oxygen, *tissue perfusion is inadequate relative to metabolic needs.*

Categorization by Severity

In addition to the severity of end-organ effects, the severity of shock is categorized by its effect on systolic blood pressure. Shock is categorized as *compensated* as long as compensatory mechanisms (eg, tachycardia, increased systemic vascular resistance) are able to maintain a normal systolic blood pressure. When compensatory mechanisms fail and systolic blood pressure drops, shock is then classified as *hypotensive* (previously referred to as *decompensated* shock).

Hypotensive shock is easy to recognize; recognition of compensated shock is more difficult. Shock may range from mild to moderate to severe. The signs and symptoms of shock are related to the type of shock and the child's compensatory responses. *Severe shock may present with normal <u>or</u> low systolic blood pressure.* In some cases children will present with low systolic blood pressure but will still meet tissue metabolic demand.

Keep in mind that automated blood pressure devices are not reliable in children with absent distal pulses and weak central pulses. Assume that these patients have hypotensive shock if other clinical signs are consistent.

Categorization of Shock by Type

Types of Shock

Shock can be categorized as follows:

Type	Description
Hypovolemic (including hemorrhagic)	Inadequate blood volume that may be complicated by inadequate oxygen-carrying capacity (ie, anemia)
Distributive (including septic, anaphylactic, neurogenic)	Inappropriately distributed blood volume and flow
Cardiogenic	Insufficient cardiac output caused by poor myocardial function
Obstructive	Obstructed blood flow—either into or out of the heart

Resources

Please read the Recognition of Shock chapter and the Management of Shock chapter in the Provider Manual.

Use of the Pediatric Assessment Approach in Evaluating Shock

Introduction

Use the systematic approach to pediatric assessment to evaluate a seriously ill or injured child for shock.

General Assessment

Look for the following signs of decreased perfusion in the initial quick visual and auditory evaluation of the child:

Appearance—The child will appear ill and may be listless with decreased response to the environment (eg, parents, caretakers, stimulation).

Work of breathing—The child may have an *increased respiratory rate* as a result of inadequate perfusion of the vital organs. For example, quiet tachypnea in a child may indicate a respiratory compensation metabolic acidosis due to tissue hypoxia. Other signs of *respiratory effort* (eg, nasal flaring, retractions) usually reflect respiratory distress and are not commonly seen in hypovolemic shock. In cardiogenic and obstructive shock, however, pulmonary edema causes increased respiratory effort, often an important component of the diagnosis. Increased respiratory effort may or may not be seen in septic shock.

Circulation—The child may have mottled or *pale, diaphoretic skin* as a result of increased vascular resistance in the peripheral circulation. *Cyanosis* can be seen with some types of cardiogenic and obstructive shock.

Primary Assessment

If you suspect shock in the seriously ill or injured child, look carefully for signs of shock during the primary assessment.

Airway

Evaluate the airway for patency. In compensated shock the airway is usually patent. As decompensation occurs, the child's level of consciousness may deteriorate, compromising the child's ability to maintain the airway. Assistance may be necessary.

Breathing

Increased respiratory rate and quiet tachypnea may be present. If the child is in decompensated shock or has pulmonary edema, breathing may be labored. Other signs of increased respiratory effort are usually indications of respiratory distress and not hypovolemic shock. Note that increased respiratory effort is commonly seen in cardiogenic and obstructive shock but may or may not be present with septic shock. Therefore, recognition of increased respiratory effort can be helpful in the initial diagnosis of these conditions.

Use pulse oximetry to measure oxyhemoglobin saturation. But if the peripheral perfusion is poor, pulse oximetry may be unsuccessful or unreliable.

Circulation

Conduct a thorough evaluation of the circulation, including both

- Cardiovascular function assessment—heart rate; blood pressure and pulse pressure; and capillary refill time
- End-organ function assessment—skin, brain, and renal perfusion

Heart Rate

Tachycardia is an important early sign of shock. Tachycardia and increased cardiac contractility are 2 compensatory mechanisms that help to maintain cardiac output during shock.

Although tachycardia is an early and sensitive indicator of shock, it is not specific to shock. There are many other causes of tachycardia, such as pain, fear, anger, and fever. If any of these noncardiac causes is responsible for the tachycardia, you should be able to easily palpate the child's distal pulses. But the child may also demonstrate tachycardia with palpable peripheral pulses during the early stages of septic shock. If peripheral pulses are absent, the tachycardia is almost always due to shock with low cardiac output and increased systemic vascular resistance.

Heart rate should decrease gradually as shock is successfully treated. But you should interpret heart rate in the context of other clinical findings. Bradycardia is a late and ominous sign.

Blood Pressure

Measure blood pressure initially and with each reassessment. Remember that automated blood pressure measurement may be unreliable when pulses are not palpable. At first compensatory mechanisms may maintain blood pressure by increasing systemic vascular resistance, causing vasoconstriction. Hypotension is a late and often sudden sign of cardiovascular decompensation. Therefore, you should treat even mild hypotension quickly and vigorously because it signals decompensation with possible imminent cardiac arrest. Hypotension may occur early in septic shock.

Pulses (Peripheral and Central) and Pulse Pressure

The femoral, brachial, radial, posterior tibial, and dorsal pedal pulses should be readily palpable in healthy infants and children. The palpable pulse volume (strength of the pulse) is normally related to stroke volume and pulse pressure (the difference between systolic and diastolic pressures).

Look for these signs of shock when palpating pulses:

Sign	Description
Narrowing pulse pressure with "thready" pulses	Pulse pressure changes as a result of decreased cardiac output and a compensatory increase in systemic vascular resistance. In shock with low cardiac output, pulse pressure will typically narrow and distal pulses may feel "thready." If cardiac output continues to fall, pulse pressure will decrease further and pulses will no longer be palpable.
Wide pulse pressure with bounding pulses	Some types of shock (such as septic shock) may be characterized by a wide pulse pressure with normal or increased stroke volume and low systemic vascular resistance, leading to bounding pulses.
Loss of peripheral and central pulses	A discrepancy in volume between peripheral and central pulses is an important sign of decreased cardiac output. Loss of central pulses indicates cardiac arrest and the need for immediate CPR.

Capillary Refill Time

Sluggish, delayed, or prolonged capillary refill (a refill time of more than 2 seconds) can be a sign of shock, fever, or cold ambient temperature. Brisk capillary refill may be present in septic shock. Interpret capillary refill in the context of other signs of shock because it is a relatively insensitive and nonspecific indicator of shock when assessed alone. Be sure to measure capillary refill with the distal extremity above the level of the heart.

Skin Perfusion

Skin color and temperature (presuming warm ambient temperature) are important clinical signs in the evaluation of systemic perfusion. The nail beds, soles of the feet, and palms of the hands should be pink. Cool extremities and pale, diaphoretic skin are early signs of shock. When cardiac output decreases, cooling of the skin can initially develop peripherally (in the fingers and toes) and then extend proximally (toward the trunk). You may be able to identify a line of demarcation between warm and cool skin.

Brain Perfusion

Observe mental status, general appearance, and response to stimulation (AVPU* Pediatric Response Scale score). Look for the following signs of inadequate brain perfusion:

- Altered level of consciousness with confusion
- Irritability
- Lethargy
- Agitation alternating with lethargy
- Decreased response to caregiver or environment

Altered mental status is one of the most important clinical indicators of deteriorating shock in a child.

***A** = **A**lert; **V** = Responsive to **V**oice; **P** = Responsive to **P**ain; **U** = **U**nresponsive

Renal Perfusion

Adequate urine output depends on adequate renal blood flow. Urine flow of less than 1 mL/kg per hour in an infant or young child or less than 30 mL per hour in adolescents in the absence of known renal disease can be an important sign of decreased systemic cardiovascular perfusion.

Remember that urine present in the bladder when a catheter is placed is not helpful in the initial evaluation of renal perfusion because it may represent urine production over various time periods. Ongoing urine output provides much better information.

Disability

The AVPU scale, the Glasgow Coma Scale, and pupillary responses can be used to monitor the child for signs of compromised brain perfusion. (See "Disability" in the Primary Assessment section.)

Exposure

You should undress ("expose" for visual exam) every seriously ill or injured child as appropriate for a thorough physical examination. Exposure often provides important information leading to the diagnosis of the underlying condition.

Look for evidence of trauma, ie, significant bleeding or other significant injury. Assess core temperature and avoid exposure hypothermia.

Recognition of Shock Flowchart

Figure 22 outlines the approach to recognizing the type and severity of shock. At any point during your evaluation, be alert to life-threatening conditions. If you identify one, intervene immediately and activate the ERS.

	Clinical Signs	Hypovolemic Shock	Distributive Shock	Cardiogenic Shock	Obstructive Shock
A	Patency	Airway open and maintainable/not maintainable			
B	Respiratory rate	Increased			
	Respiratory effort	Normal to increased		Labored	
	Breath sounds	Normal	Normal (± crackles)	Crackles, grunting	
C	Systolic blood pressure	**Compensated Shock ➡ Hypotensive Shock**			
	Pulse pressure	Narrow	Wide	Narrow	
	Heart rate	Increased			
	Peripheral pulse quality	Weak	Bounding or weak	Weak	
	Skin	Pale, cool	Warm or cool	Pale, cool	
	Capillary refill	Delayed	Variable	Delayed	
	Urine output	Decreased			
D	Level of consciousness	Irritable early Lethargic late			
E	Temperature	Variable			

Figure 22. Recognition of Shock Flowchart

Fundamentals of Shock Management

Management of Shock Emergencies Flowchart

Figure 23 outlines general management of shock and specific management according to the type of circulatory problem. Please note that this chart does not include all circulatory emergencies; it provides key management strategies for a limited number of conditions.

Management of Shock Emergencies Flowchart

- Oxygen
- Pulse oximetry
- ECG monitor
- IV/IO access
- BLS as indicated
- Bedside glucose

Hypovolemic Shock
Specific Management for Selected Conditions

Nonhemorrhagic	*Hemorrhagic*
• 20 mL/kg NS/LR bolus, repeat as needed • Consider colloid after 3rd NS/LR bolus	• Control external bleeding • 20 mL/kg NS/LR bolus repeat 2 or 3× as needed • Transfuse PRBCs as indicated

Distributive Shock
Specific Management for Selected Conditions

Septic	*Anaphylactic*	*Neurogenic*
Management Algorithm: • Septic Shock	• IM epinephrine (or auto-injector) • Antihistamines • Corticosteroids • Epinephrine infusion • Albuterol	• 20 mL/kg NS/LR bolus, repeat PRN • Vasopressor

Cardiogenic Shock
Specific Management for Selected Conditions

Bradyarrhythmia/Tachyarrhythmia	*Other (eg, CHD, Myocarditis, Cardiomyopathy, Poisoning)*
Management Algorithms: • Bradycardia • Tachycardia with poor perfusion	• 5 to 10 mL/kg NS/LR bolus, repeat PRN • Vasoactive infusion • Consider expert consultation

Obstructive Shock
Specific Management for Selected Conditions

Ductal-Dependent *(LV Outflow Obstruction)*	*Tension Pneumothorax*	*Cardiac Tamponade*	*Pulmonary Embolism*
• Prostaglandin E_1 • Expert consultation	• Needle decompression • Tube thoracostomy	• Pericardiocentesis • 20 mL/kg NS/LR bolus	• 20 mL/kg NS/LR bolus, repeat PRN • Consider thrombolytics, anticoagulants • Expert consultation

Figure 23. Management of Shock Emergencies Flowchart.

Guidelines for Fluid Therapy and Glucose

Fluid Therapy
Volume and Rate of Fluid Administration

Start fluid resuscitation for hypovolemic and distributive shock with 20 mL/kg of isotonic crystalloid (NS or LR) administered as a bolus over 5 to 20 minutes. Then administer repeat boluses of 20 mL/kg as needed to restore blood pressure and perfusion. Adjust the rate of fluid according to the underlying cause of shock. Smaller fluid boluses (5 to 10 mL/kg) given more slowly are used if indicated in cardiogenic shock. In obstructive shock other therapies are often indicated rather than fluid administration (eg, needle decompression of a pneumothorax). Small fluid boluses can also be used to temporize cardiac tamponade until it can be relieved.

Do not use glucose in these bolus fluids.

Indication for Blood Products

Blood and blood products are not the first choice for immediate volume expansion in children with shock. Blood is recommended for replacement of volume loss in pediatric trauma victims with inadequate perfusion despite administration of 2 to 3 boluses of 20 mL/kg of isotonic crystalloid. Under these circumstances packed red blood cells (PRBCs) 10 mL/kg should then be administered as soon as available.

Priorities for transfusion include the following blood products in order:

- Crossmatched
- Type-specific
- Type O*

*Type O negative for girls and either negative or positive for boys

Glucose
Diagnosis of Hypoglycemia

Blood glucose monitoring is important in shock management. Hypoglycemia is a common finding in seriously ill children, and it can result in brain injury if it is not recognized and effectively treated.

Use the lowest acceptable glucose concentrations to define hypoglycemia:

Age	Consensus Definition of Hypoglycemia
Preterm neonates Term neonates	≤45 mg/dL
Infants Children Adolescents	≤60 mg/dL

Management of Hypoglycemia

If the glucose concentration is low and the child is alert, you may give glucose orally (eg, orange juice or other glucose-containing fluid). If the child has decreased response or is unstable, you should administer the glucose intravenously (dextrose). IV dextrose is commonly administered as $D_{25}W$ using 2 to 4 mL/kg or $D_{10}W$ using 5 to 10 mL/kg (0.5 to 1 g/kg). Reassess serum glucose concentration after giving dextrose. Establish a continuous IV infusion of dextrose-containing fluids as needed to prevent recurrence of hypoglycemia.

Do not infuse dextrose-containing fluids for volume resuscitation in shock. Bolus administration of these fluids may cause hyperglycemia, rise in serum osmolality, and osmotic diuresis exacerbating hypovolemia and shock.

PALS Septic Shock Algorithm

Study the PALS Septic Shock Algorithm (Figure 24) to prepare for the course. You may be presented with a septic shock scenario during the case simulations and core case tests. For a complete explanation of this algorithm, see the Management of Shock chapter in the Provider Manual.

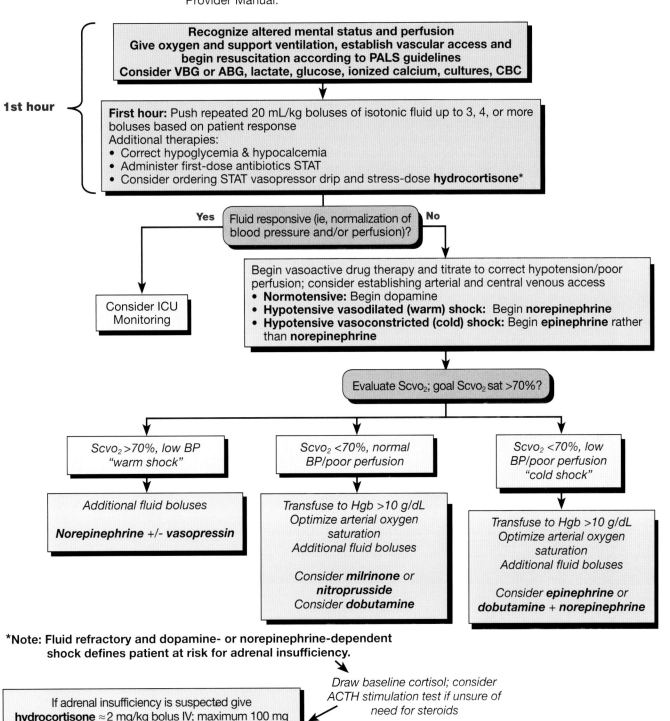

1st hour

Recognize altered mental status and perfusion
Give oxygen and support ventilation, establish vascular access and begin resuscitation according to PALS guidelines
Consider VBG or ABG, lactate, glucose, ionized calcium, cultures, CBC

First hour: Push repeated 20 mL/kg boluses of isotonic fluid up to 3, 4, or more boluses based on patient response
Additional therapies:
- Correct hypoglycemia & hypocalcemia
- Administer first-dose antibiotics STAT
- Consider ordering STAT vasopressor drip and stress-dose **hydrocortisone***

Yes ← Fluid responsive (ie, normalization of blood pressure and/or perfusion)? → **No**

Consider ICU Monitoring

Begin vasoactive drug therapy and titrate to correct hypotension/poor perfusion; consider establishing arterial and central venous access
- **Normotensive:** Begin dopamine
- **Hypotensive vasodilated (warm) shock:** Begin **norepinephrine**
- **Hypotensive vasoconstricted (cold) shock:** Begin **epinephrine** rather than **norepinephrine**

Evaluate $Scvo_2$; goal $Scvo_2$ sat >70%?

$Scvo_2$ >70%, low BP "warm shock"

$Scvo_2$ <70%, normal BP/poor perfusion

$Scvo_2$ <70%, low BP/poor perfusion "cold shock"

Additional fluid boluses
Norepinephrine +/- vasopressin

Transfuse to Hgb >10 g/dL
Optimize arterial oxygen saturation
Additional fluid boluses
Consider **milrinone** or **nitroprusside**
Consider **dobutamine**

Transfuse to Hgb >10 g/dL
Optimize arterial oxygen saturation
Additional fluid boluses
Consider **epinephrine** or **dobutamine + norepinephrine**

*Note: Fluid refractory and dopamine- or norepinephrine-dependent shock defines patient at risk for adrenal insufficiency.

Draw baseline cortisol; consider ACTH stimulation test if unsure of need for steroids

If adrenal insufficiency is suspected give **hydrocortisone** ≈2 mg/kg bolus IV; maximum 100 mg

Modified from Parker MM, Hazelzet JA, Carcillo JA. Pediatric considerations. Crit Care Med. 2004;32:S591-S594.

Figure 24. PALS Septic Shock Algorithm.

Drugs Used in Shock Management

Summary

The following drugs may be used in shock management:

- Albuterol
- Alprostadil
- Calcium chloride
- Corticosteroids
- Dextrose (Glucose)
- Dobutamine
- Dopamine
- Epinephrine
- Norepinephrine
- Milrinone
- Nitroglycerin
- Sodium nitroprusside
- Vasopressin

See the Management of Shock chapter in the Provider Manual for a discussion of drug selection based on the cardiovascular physiology according to type of shock.

See Part 10: Pharmacology for indications and dosing.

Shock Learning Station Competency Checklists 1-4

Shock Core Case 1 Hypovolemic Shock	Use this checklist during the PALS core case simulations and tests to check off the performance of the team leader.
Critical Performance Steps	**Details**
Team Leader	
___ **Assigns team member roles**	Team leader identifies self and assigns team roles
___ **Uses effective communication throughout**	Closed-loop communication Clear messages Clear roles and responsibilities Knowing one's limitations Knowledge sharing Constructive intervention Reevaluation and summarizing Mutual respect
Patient Management	
___ **Directs assessment of airway, breathing, circulation, disability, and exposure, including vital signs**	Team leader directs or performs assessment to determine airway patency, adequacy of breathing and circulation, level of responsiveness, temperature, and vital signs
___ **Directs administration of 100% oxygen**	Team leader directs administration of 100% oxygen
___ **Directs placement of pads/leads and pulse oximetry**	Team leader directs that pads/leads be properly placed and that the monitor be turned on to an appropriate lead; requests use of pulse oximetry
___ **Recognizes signs and symptoms of hypovolemic shock**	Team leader verbalizes features of history and exam that indicate hypovolemic shock
___ **Categorizes as compensated or hypotensive shock**	Team leader verbalizes whether patient is compensated or hypotensive
___ **Directs IV or IO access**	Team leader directs team member to place IO (or IV) line; line placement simulated properly
___ **Directs rapid administration of a fluid bolus of isotonic crystalloid**	Team leader directs administration of isotonic crystalloid, 20 mL/kg rapidly IV or IO
___ **Directs reassessment of patient in response to treatment**	Team leader directs team members to reassess airway, breathing, and circulation
Case Conclusion	
___ **Verbalizes therapeutic end points during shock management**	Team leader identifies parameters that indicate response to therapy (heart rate, blood pressure, distal pulses and capillary refill, urine output, mental status)

Shock Core Case 2 Obstructive Shock	Use this checklist during the PALS core case simulations and tests to check off the performance of the team leader.
Critical Performance Steps	**Details**

Team Leader

___ **Assigns team member roles**	Team leader identifies self and assigns team roles
___ **Uses effective communication throughout**	Closed-loop communication Clear messages Clear roles and responsibilities Knowing one's limitations Knowledge sharing Constructive intervention Reevaluation and summarizing Mutual respect

Patient Management

___ **Directs assessment of airway, breathing, circulation, disability, and exposure, including vital signs**	Team leader directs or performs assessment to determine airway patency, adequacy of breathing and circulation, level of responsiveness, temperature, and vital signs
___ **Directs placement of pads/leads and pulse oximetry**	Team leader directs that pads/leads be properly placed and that the monitor be turned on to an appropriate lead; requests use of pulse oximetry
___ **Verbalizes "DOPE" mnemonic for intubated patient who deteriorates**	Team leader reviews elements of DOPE mnemonic (displacement, obstruction, pneumothorax, equipment failure + gastric distention)
___ **Recognizes signs and symptoms of obstructive shock**	Team leader verbalizes features of history and exam that indicate obstructive shock
___ **States at least 2 causes of obstructive shock**	Team leader states at least 2 common causes of obstructive shock (tension pneumothorax, cardiac tamponade, pulmonary embolus)
___ **Categorizes as compensated or hypotensive shock**	Team leader verbalizes whether patient is compensated or hypotensive
___ **Directs IV or IO access**	Team leader directs team member to place IO (or IV) line; line placement simulated properly
___ **Directs rapid administration of a fluid bolus of isotonic crystalloid**	Team leader directs administration of isotonic crystalloid, 20 mL/kg rapidly IV or IO
___ **Directs reassessment of patient in response to treatment**	Team leader directs team member to reassess airway, breathing, and circulation

Case Conclusion

___ **Summarizes the treatment for a tension pneumothorax**	Team leader describes use of emergency pleural decompression (second intercostal space, midclavicular line)
___ **Verbalizes therapeutic end points during shock management**	Team leader identifies parameters that indicate response to therapy (heart rate, blood pressure, perfusion, urine output, mental status)

Shock Core Case 3 Distributive (Septic) Shock	*Use this checklist during the PALS core case simulations and tests to check off the performance of the team leader.*
Critical Performance Steps	**Details**
___ **Assigns team member roles**	Team leader identifies self and assigns team roles
Team Leader	
___ **Uses effective communication throughout**	Closed-loop communication Clear messages Clear roles and responsibilities Knowing one's limitations Knowledge sharing Constructive intervention Reevaluation and summarizing Mutual respect
Patient Management	
___ **Directs assessment of airway, breathing, circulation, disability, and exposure, including vital signs**	Team leader directs or performs assessment to determine airway patency, adequacy of breathing and circulation, level of responsiveness, temperature, and vital signs
___ **Directs administration of 100% oxygen**	Team leader directs team member to provide 100% oxygen
___ **Directs placement of pads/leads and pulse oximetry**	Team leader directs that pads/leads be properly placed and that the monitor be turned on to an appropriate lead; requests use of pulse oximetry
___ **Recognizes signs and symptoms of distributive (septic) shock**	Team leader verbalizes features of history and exam that indicate distributive shock
___ **Categorizes as compensated or hypotensive shock**	Team leader verbalizes whether patient is compensated or hypotensive
___ **Directs IV or IO access**	Team leader directs team member to place IO (or IV) line; line placement simulated properly
___ **Directs rapid administration of a fluid bolus of isotonic crystalloid**	Team leader directs administration of isotonic crystalloid, 20 mL/kg rapidly IV or IO
___ **Directs reassessment of patient in response to treatment**	Team leader directs team member to reassess airway, breathing, and circulation
___ ***If scope of practice applies:* Recalls that early administration of antibiotics is essential in septic shock**	*If scope of practice applies:* Team leader directs administration of antibiotics
Case Conclusion	
___ **Summarizes indications for vasoactive drug support**	Team leader verbalizes that vasoactive medications are indicated for fluid-refractory septic shock
___ **Verbalizes therapeutic end points during shock management**	Team leader identifies parameters that indicate response to therapy (heart rate, blood pressure, perfusion, urine output, mental status)

Shock Core Case 4 Cardiogenic Shock	Use this checklist during the PALS core case simulations and tests to check off the performance of the team leader.
Critical Performance Steps	**Details**
___ Assigns team member roles	Team leader identifies self and assigns team roles
Team Leader	
___ Uses effective communication throughout	Closed-loop communication Clear messages Clear roles and responsibilities Knowing one's limitations Knowledge sharing Constructive intervention Reevaluation and summarizing Mutual respect
Patient Management	
___ Directs assessment of airway, breathing, circulation, disability, and exposure, including vital signs	Team leader directs or performs assessment to determine responsiveness, breathing, and pulse
___ Directs administration of 100% oxygen	Team leader directs administration of 100% oxygen by high-flow device
___ Directs placement of pads/leads and pulse oximetry	Team leader directs that pads/leads be properly placed and that the monitor be turned on to an appropriate lead; requests use of pulse oximetry
___ Recognizes signs and symptoms of cardiogenic shock	Team leader verbalizes features of history and exam that indicate cardiogenic shock
___ Categorizes as compensated or hypotensive shock	Team leader verbalizes whether patient's shock is compensated or hypotensive (previously referred to as decompensated shock)
___ Directs IV or IO access	Team leader directs team member to place IO (or IV) line; line placement simulated properly
___ Directs slow administration of a 10 mL/kg fluid bolus of isotonic crystalloid	Team leader directs administration of isotonic crystalloid, 10 mL/kg IV or IO, while carefully monitoring patient for signs of pulmonary edema or worsening heart failure
___ Directs reassessment of the patient in response to treatment	Team leader directs team member to reassess airway, breathing, and circulation
___ Recalls indications for use of vasoactive drugs during cardiogenic shock	Team leader verbalizes indications for initiation of vasoactive drugs (poor response to fluid therapy, persistent hypotension)
Case Conclusion	
___ Verbalizes therapeutic end points during shock management	Team leader identifies parameters that indicate response to therapy (heart rate, blood pressure, perfusion, urine output, mental status). In cardiogenic shock, team leader recognizes importance of reducing metabolic demand by reducing work of breathing and temperature.

Part 10

Pharmacology

Drug	Indications/Dosage
Adenosine	**SVT** 0.1 mg/kg IV/IO *rapid* push (max 6 mg), 2nd dose 0.2 mg/kg IV/IO *rapid* push (max 12 mg)
Albumin	**Shock, Trauma, Burns** 0.5 to 1 g/kg (10 to 20 mL/kg of 5% solution) IV/IO *rapid* infusion
Albuterol	**Asthma, Anaphylaxis (bronchospasm), Hyperkalemia** • MDI: 4 to 8 puffs INH q 20 minutes PRN with spacer (OR ET if intubated) • Nebulizer: 2.5 mg/dose (wt <20 kg) OR 5 mg/dose (wt >20 kg) INH q 20 minutes PRN • Continuous nebulizer: 0.5 mg/kg per hour INH (max 20 mg/h)
Alprostadil (PGE1)	**Ductal-dependent Congenital Heart Disease (all forms)** 0.05 to 0.1 µg/kg per minute IV/IO infusion initially, then 0.01 to 0.05 µg/kg per minute IV/IO
Amiodarone	**SVT, VT (with pulses)** 5 mg/kg IV/IO *load* over 20 to 60 min (max 300 mg), repeat to daily max 15 mg/kg (or 2.2 g) **Pulseless Arrest (ie, VF/pulseless VT)** 5 mg/kg IV/IO *bolus* (max 300 mg), repeat to daily max 15 mg/kg (or 2.2 g)
Atropine sulfate	**Bradycardia (symptomatic)** • 0.02 mg/kg IV/IO (min dose 0.1 mg, max single dose child 0.5 mg, max single dose adolescent 1 mg), may repeat dose once, max total dose child 1 mg, max total dose adolescent 2 mg • 0.04 to 0.06 mg/kg ET **Toxins/Overdose (eg, organophosphate, carbamate)** 0.02 to 0.05 mg/kg (<12 years) OR 0.05 mg/kg (>12 years) IV/IO initially, repeat q 20 to 30 min until atropine effect (dry mouth, tachycardia, mydriasis) is observed or symptoms reverse
Calcium chloride 10%	**Hypocalcemia, Hyperkalemia, Hypermagnesemia, Calcium Channel Blocker Overdose** 20 mg/kg (0.2 mL/kg) IV/IO *slow* push during arrest or if severe hypotension, repeat PRN
Dexamethasone	**Croup** 0.6 mg/kg PO/IM/IV (max 16 mg)
Dextrose (Glucose)	**Hypoglycemia** 0.5 to 1 g/kg IV/IO ($D_{25}W$ 2 to 4 mL/kg; $D_{10}W$ 5 to 10 mL/kg)
Diphenhydramine	**Anaphylactic Shock** 1 to 2 mg/kg IV/IO/IM q 4 to 6 hours (max 50 mg)
Dobutamine	**Congestive Heart Failure, Cardiogenic Shock** 2 to 20 µg/kg per minute IV/IO infusion; titrate to desired effect

Drug	Indications/Dosage
Dopamine	**Cardiogenic Shock, Distributive Shock** 2 to 20 µg/kg per minute IV/IO infusion; titrate to desired effect
Epinephrine	**Pulseless Arrest, Bradycardia (symptomatic)** • 0.01 mg/kg (0.1 mL/kg) 1:10 000 IV/IO q 3 to 5 minutes (max 1 mg; 1 mL) • 0.1 mg/kg (0.1 mL/kg) 1:1000 ET q 3 to 5 minutes **Hypotensive Shock** 0.1 to 1 µg/kg per minute IV/IO infusion (consider higher doses if needed) **Anaphylaxis** • 0.01 mg/kg (0.01 mL/kg) 1:1000 IM in thigh q 15 minutes PRN (max 0.5 mg) OR • Auto-injector 0.3 mg (wt ≥30 kg) IM or Child Jr auto-injector 0.15 mg (wt 10 to 30 kg) IM • 0.01 mg/kg (0.1 mL/kg) 1:10 000 IV/IO q 3 to 5 minutes (max 1 mg) if hypotension • 0.1 to 1 µg/kg per minute IV/IO infusion if hypotension despite fluids and IM injection **Asthma** 0.01 mg/kg (0.01 mL/kg) 1:1000 SQ q 15 minutes (max 0.5 mg; 0.5 mL) **Croup** 0.25 to 0.5 mL *racemic* solution (2.25%) mixed in 3 mL NS INH OR 3 mL 1:1000 INH **Toxins/Overdose (eg, β-adrenergic blocker, calcium channel blocker)** • 0.01 mg/kg (0.1 mL/kg) 1:10 000 IV/IO (max 1 mg); if no response consider higher doses up to 0.1 mg/kg (0.1 mL/kg) 1:1000 IV/IO • 0.1 to 1 µg/kg per minute IV/IO infusion (consider higher doses)
Furosemide	**Pulmonary Edema, Fluid Overload** 1 mg/kg IV/IM (usual max 20 mg if not chronically on loop diuretic)
Hydrocortisone	**Adrenal Insufficiency** 2 mg/kg IV bolus (max 100 mg)
Inamrinone	**Myocardial Dysfunction and Increased SVR/PVR** Loading dose: 0.75 to 1 mg/kg IV/IO slow bolus over 5 minutes (may repeat twice to max 3 mg/kg), then 5 to 10 µg/kg per minute IV/IO infusion
Ipratropium bromide	**Asthma** 250 to 500 µg INH q 20 minutes PRN × 3 doses
Lidocaine	**VF/Pulseless VT, Wide-Complex Tachycardia (with pulses)** • 1 mg/kg IV/IO bolus • Maintenance: 20 to 50 µg/kg per minute IV/IO infusion (repeat bolus dose if infusion initiated >15 minutes, after initial bolus) • 2 to 3 mg/kg ET
Magnesium sulfate	**Asthma (refractory status asthmaticus), Torsades de Pointes, Hypomagnesemia** 25 to 50 mg/kg IV/IO *bolus* (pulseless VT) OR over 10 to 20 minutes (VT with pulses) OR *slow* infusion over 15 to 30 minutes (status asthmaticus); (max 2 g)
Methylprednisolone	**Asthma (status asthmaticus), Anaphylactic Shock** • Load: 2 mg/kg IV/IO/IM (max 80 mg); use acetate salt IM • Maintenance: 0.5 mg/kg IV/IO q 6 hours (max 120 mg/d)
Milrinone	**Myocardial Dysfunction and Increased SVR/PVR** Loading dose: 50 to 75 µg/kg IV/IO over 10 to 60 minutes followed by 0.5 to 0.75 µg/kg per minute IV/IO infusion

Drug	Indications/Dosage
Naloxone	**Narcotic (opiate) Reversal** • Total reversal required (for narcotic toxicity secondary to overdose): 0.1 mg/kg IV/IO/IM/SQ bolus q 2 minutes PRN (max 2 mg) • Total reversal not required (eg, for respiratory depression associated with therapeutic narcotic use): 1 to 5 µg/kg IV/IO/IM/SQ; titrate to desired effect • Maintain reversal: 0.002 to 0.16 mg/kg per hour IV/IO infusion
Nitroglycerin	**Congestive Heart Failure, Cardiogenic Shock** • 0.25 to 0.5 µg/kg per minute IV/IO infusion, may increase by 0.5 to 1 µg/kg per minute q 3 to 5 minutes PRN to 1 to 5 µg/kg per minute (max 10 µg/kg per minute) • Adolescents: 10 to 20 µg/min, increase by 5 to 10 µg/min every 5 to 10 minutes PRN to max 200 µg/min
Norepinephrine	**Hypotensive (usually distributive) Shock (ie, low SVR and fluid refractory)** 0.1 to 2 µg/kg per minute IV/IO infusion; titrate to desired effect
Oxygen	**Hypoxia, Hypoxemia, Shock, Trauma, Cardiopulmonary Failure, Cardiac Arrest** Administer 100% O_2 via high-flow O_2 delivery system (if spontaneous ventilations) or ET (if intubated); titrate to desired effect
Procainamide	**SVT, Atrial Flutter, VT (with pulses)** 15 mg/kg IV/IO load over 30 to 60 minutes (do not use routinely with amiodarone)
Sodium bicarbonate	**Metabolic Acidosis (severe), Hyperkalemia** 1 mEq/kg IV/IO *slow* bolus **Sodium Channel Blocker Overdose (eg, tricyclic antidepressant)** 1 to 2 mEq/kg IV/IO bolus until serum pH is >7.45 (7.50 to 7.55 for severe overdose) followed by IV/IO infusion of 150 mEq $NaHCO_3$/L solution to maintain alkalosis
Sodium nitroprusside	**Cardiogenic Shock (ie, associated with high SVR), Severe Hypertension** 1 to 8 µg/kg per minute (wt <40 kg) OR 0.1 to 5 µg/kg per minute (wt >40 kg) IV/IO infusion
Terbutaline	**Asthma (status asthmaticus), Hyperkalemia** • 0.1 to 10 µg/kg per minute IV/IO infusion; consider 10 µg/kg IV/IO load over 5 minutes • 10 µg/kg SQ q 10 to 15 minutes until IV/IO infusion is initiated (max 0.4 mg)